How To Look Years You

Contents

Introduction

Most people that meet me assume that I am in my early to mid forties. They are surprised when I tell them that I am in fact already 60. Over the last 15 to 20 years, many friends, colleagues and others have asked me what I have done to look so youthful – what is my secret? What surgery must I have undergone? What pills must I be taking? Which creams am I applying? I used to answer that it is none of these but that I do have some 'secrets' and one day I will put them into a book for others to use. Indeed there are a few things that I have done for a large part of my life that almost certainly have contributed to the younger looking me. So, for those people that I promised and to millions of others who undoubtedly also wish to look younger, I have finally 'put pen to paper'.

Some so-called experts will claim that I have just been lucky with my genes. This might be believable if it were just one aspect but cannot account for so many areas such as skin, hair, health, face, feet, posture, weight, teeth and so on; the combination of which contribute to how young a person looks. All of these different features and more will be addressed in this book – I will explain things that I do (and have done for some time) which keep all of these areas youthful. Genetics seems to be a current scientific excuse for so many things from over-weight to ill-health and state of mind. Male pattern baldness for example was supposed to be genetic on your father's side (through to your grandfather). Suddenly, research suggests it might be from your mother's genes. As usual, the experts don't seem to agree. But one thing is for sure and that is if you want to achieve something then a well tried approach is simply to copy a person who is already successful in that area.

Some of these techniques that I will describe are simply a way of carrying out things that the majority of people do every day but differently. Most of them take me no extra time at all. It is just that I have discovered ways of doing certain things which I believe have contributed to my overall more youthful appearance; even things as simple as how you brush your hair. All you have to do is copy these methods to obtain similar results. There are those that suggest that aging is a natural phenomenon and therefore it should be accepted as the natural order of things. While it may be true that aging is normal, that doesn't make everything about it desirable! On the other hand, not everything about aging is bad news and we shall consider some of these good points too. I hear that the best spouse a person can have is an archaeologist because the older you get, the more interested they become!

A few of the things described in this book will take a little extra time to do, such as certain exercises that I carry out either daily or every few days. However most of these only take a few minutes to complete and after a while they will become second nature for you, as they have for me.

None of my revelations are based on using some magic potion or cream. Furthermore there really is no need to have plastic surgery when these simple techniques exist that clearly work and are free and natural. They have no risk, are not painful and cannot end up with some of the disasters you hear of with cosmetic surgery. Not only will you look great but you will also feel better. However, it is not good enough just reading this book and hoping that the knowledge alone will have an effect; you will have to take action. Somebody once said "For things to change in your life, first you must change yourself" I suspect it is based on this quote supposedly from Gandhi - "**you** must be the change you wish to see in the world."

As I am a male, there might be a few things in this book which are specific to males and though not deliberately, perhaps it will have been written rather from a male perspective but I can assure you that the majority of what I am about to reveal is relevant to both men and women.

So let's start at the top of your head and work our way down your body as well as discuss a variety of other subjects, all to help you look at least 10 years younger and all naturally!

While you are reading, keep in mind these words attributed to Mae West -
"You're never too old to become younger."

Chapter 1 - Your Hair

Although our hair seems to have no biological use any more, it has an enormous social symbolism and significance in terms of beauty, health and youthfulness. What things do I carry out with my hair and just as importantly, perhaps, what things do I avoid which seem to have resulted in my still having a full head of hair which is thick and healthy? We'll look at the use of combs (or the abuse of these), massage, all those wonder products, exercise, addressing greying hair and a heap of other subjects. It would be wonderful if everybody could have hair that grew strongly and vigorously, wouldn't it? Hopefully your hair is your crowning glory! If it is then perhaps you should start now to take note of this chapter to ensure it stays that way. If not, well use these simple approaches and let me know the results and improvements that you find occurring.

Like most teenagers I was quite obsessed about my appearance. I was frequently looking in the mirror and combing my hair. I don't know about nowadays but back then it was common to carry a comb in your back pocket. One day I was horrified to discover that my hair seemed to be receding – I was developing the classic "widow's peak". After many weeks seeing the situation worsening, I started to give the problem much thought. I concluded that the culprit was my comb – firstly that it was dragging the hair too hard and secondly that scratching it over my scalp probably wasn't too good for my hair follicles either.

I decided right then and there that I would throw out all of my combs and from then onwards, I have only ever used my "God-given comb" – my fingers. Not only has this been cheaper but it meant I have always had a comb to hand (excuse the pun). More importantly, my hair stopped receding and as you can see, I still have a very strong hairline – the same one that I had as a teenager after I stopped using a comb. By the way, I do not use a hair brush either, I only use my fingers to put my hair in place – I hold them about a centimetre apart and use them like a comb. It might sound impossible for those of you who spend ages in front of a mirror with brushes and combs of various sorts but after you get the hang of it, it works perfectly. One hint is to make sure your fingers are dry if your hair is wet. I wear my hair with a parting to one side but to avoid the possibility of habitually dragging my hair in the same place, I usually part it somewhere else while I am initially smoothing out my hair then arrange it in its regular position last of all. Another thing about too much combing and brushing is that it could wear away the hairs' cuticles (its protective outer layer). This could end up catching on other hairs, causing tangles. If the cuticle were further worn down, the inner cortex could be exposed, seriously weakening the hair. The final result could be split ends. Now I realise that some of you might have quite long beautiful hair and perhaps the only way to control it is to use a comb or brush but I would suggest that you consider using one with wide apart, soft, rounded, thick teeth. Remember what Oliver Herford, the American humorist apparently said – "A hair in the head is worth two in the brush." But there was another very important outcome of using my fingers and that was that I was effectively massaging my scalp as I 'brushed' my hair and I believe that this is extremely important in developing healthy, strong, shiny, vigorously growing hair.

In fact, when I wash my hair, I actually view it as a scalp massage, not a hair shampooing. This is a technique you should think about developing in order to improve the quality of your hair and also to keep it growing strongly – I am not thinning at all and I believe that this is in large part due to the fact that I massage my head in the shower instead of just washing my hair. One of the main benefits of massage is to improve blood circulation and this is certainly important as far as your scalp, hair follicles and pores are concerned. Such massage also spreads the natural oils of the hair, increasing hair lustre. It also encourages nourishment to be sent to the capillary vessels in hair papillae which activates the hair cells. I have been doing this for many years and it is interesting that I read an article quite recently that claimed that there were ancient Chinese scalp massage techniques that would stop you thinning or going bald. Apparently Indian Ayervedic head massage has also been around for thousands of years. You might be intrigued to learn that 'Champi' is the Indian word for "head massage" and is the origin of the English word shampoo. Well, what I do is massage all over my scalp very firmly with my finger tips and thumb tips (note – do not use your fingernails!), including, for me as a male, right down my sideburns. This only takes two or three minutes – probably no longer than simply washing your hair. Now, since I have never thinned, I cannot guarantee this but I would not be surprised if massaging in this way would help stop thinning or even help re-growth – let me know how you go. While you are at it, you might as well spend another minute or two massaging the back of your neck down to your shoulders – this is a great stress reliever and a wonderful start to the day! A double benefit is that reducing stress helps improve circulation and hair growth. By the way, if you want to do your loved ones including your children a favour, you could learn to give this sort of head and neck massage to others.

Whenever I go to the hairdresser's, they invariably tell me what thick, strong hair I have and how quickly it grows. They often tell me how lucky I am and I agree – however, the only luck is to have discovered a few things which I am now doing regularly to keep my hair so healthy. For example, the only time a hairdryer is ever used on me is at the hairdresser's, otherwise I never employ one myself. I'm sure it cannot be good for your hair and even worse for your scalp, especially if it is too hot. Those of you who have very long hair perhaps feel you have no option but please avoid burning your scalp and over-heating your hair. Perhaps one way to avoid heat damage would be to keep your hairdryer or alternatively your hair moving. Apart from towelling, the main way I dry my hair is by squeezing and gently pulling my hand down the hair shaft. This also means that I am pulling my hair somewhat which reminds me of the technique of hair pulling I have heard of to make your hair strong. However, I would sound a word of caution here; I am not recommending that you actually pull hard on your hair which could lead to follicle damage!

There's another thing which I've often speculated about whether it has helped – although I like hats and sometimes wear them, it is quite infrequent. I wonder if continuous wearing of hats contributes to poor hair. It has been suggested that they cause bad circulation, which could deprive the hair of proper nutrition. Build up of sweat, dirt, and grime around the rim probably also creates follicle ill-health. It would be interesting to research this.

I have a general aversion to hair products – I don't particularly like the thought of all those chemicals being poured on my head. At hairdressers, they always ask what would I like on my hair and seem surprised when I say "nothing, I prefer it to be natural, thank you". I try to avoid patronising those disgusting smelling hairdressers – they reek like a chemical factory. I can't imagine the damage being done to the clients' hair! I don't even use conditioners much – perhaps once a month at most. Sure, if you feel it's the only way to prevent your long hair tangling then perhaps use a minimal amount, otherwise, I personally would suggest avoid using it too often. There's been a lot of discussion even about how bad most shampoos are for you because they contain particularly nasty chemicals such as those apparently used to degrease engines! Natural oils are clearly very important for the health of your hair and lots of hair products, including many shampoos, are almost certainly responsible for stripping these from your hair. I must say that I have always tried to give my head a rest from shampoo every so often, say once a week or so – I call it a shampoo fallow day. Some people try to replace lost natural oils by applying creams but these can apparently clog up your pores causing all sorts of problems. It might be better not to dry out your hair with chemicals and heat in the first place.

Only you can make your own decisions about the potential dangers of the many petrochemicals found in most shampoos and cosmetics. There is plenty of information to be found but for example, according to a 1995 U.S. government study they can be absorbed through the skin (including the scalp) and accumulate in the organs and tissues. This can result in brain, nerve, and liver damage. One of the most common of these toxic compounds is DEA (diethanolamine). It is formulated in hundreds of home and personal care products. This study showed that DEA has significant cumulative toxicity since it cannot be excreted from the body easily and builds up in the fatty tissues of the liver, kidneys and brain. This can lead to nerve damage and premature death. As a sceptic, I have to say that I suspect these studies were done on rats or mice so their relevance to humans is unclear. Also, such reports of studies rarely indicate what actual doses were used (and they are usually considerably higher than normal use).

While talking about the quality of your hair, let's just mention dandruff – obviously something you want to avoid. I've noticed a couple of things that seem to encourage it and so personally avoid. Firstly, I have found it very important to thoroughly rinse all the shampoo out of your hair. If you don't, it seems to cause dandruff. For this reason, it is definitely better to wash your hair in the shower and not in a sink. Secondly, if you travel much and use a lot of different hotel shampoos, this seems to lead to dandruff. Whether it's cheap and nasty shampoo or too many different formulations over a period of time I don't know but it would certainly be worth taking your own shampoo with you. Scalp infections are clearly not going to be beneficial to your hair and are best avoided by not only practicing good personal hygiene but also by not sharing hair accessories including hair brushes or combs (if you must use them at all!) and hats.

There is a technique I've often heard mentioned that is supposed to strengthen your hair and avoid its loss. In fact, I remember a kid at school who was always teased because his parents insisted on giving him a crewcut, that is, cutting his hair very short. The theory was that in some way, this would strengthen his hair. Well I have to say that it seems to be an old wive's tale – I met him many years later and he was going bald. Personally, I have always preferred longish hair styles.

However, there is a very different technique that I do practice regularly. It is part of a series of exercises that I carry out every morning and will describe in detail later but I will mention the action related to hair right now. Increasing the blood flow to the follicles could improve just about everything about your hair including its shine, health and colour, so here's what I do –

Make sure your hair is loose and bend from the waist (keeping your knees slightly bent to avoid back pain) and allow your head to hang loosely for 10-20 seconds. Then flick your hair with your fingers touching your scalp and start banging your head gently all over to encourage the blood to flow. Do this for a further 10-20 seconds or so.

One subject that we will come across frequently throughout this book is that of meditation and affirmations. There is a special chapter devoted to it but just to mention here in this chapter about hair that the meditational state is often referred to as the alpha brain-wave state. One place that people tend to go into alpha fairly easily and naturally is in the shower. So, while you are washing your hair (that is, massaging your scalp) it is a perfect time, instead of aimlessly daydreaming, to concentrate on your scalp and hair and repeat affirmations to yourself (or more importantly to your subconscious). It is also useful while in a meditational state to visualise your hair follicles and see them functioning perfectly and providing all the nutrients necessary for healthy hair. Some affirmations you might use are "my hair is growing strongly and vigorously" and "all my hair is a natural dark brown colour (or whatever colour is appropriate!!)".

This brings us to the important subject of grey hair, obviously a condition much associated with age. Most people over the age of 40 are likely to be concerned about going grey and I would assume that most people associate grey hair with older age. It is intriguing therefore that in a study of females, most actually considered greying hair on a man to be 'sexy'! It has certainly long been considered (again the good news is for males) that greying at the temples is distinguished. That said, I confess that many years ago I decided that I had to do something about the grey hairs that were appearing in my locks, so I started pulling them out. However, as the number grew, I started to think that pulling them out was probably not such a good idea since it might soon end up being a reason for thinning hair! So I devised a more clever scheme – I started cutting the individual grey hairs. This kept them out of sight but continued to keep a full head of hair. This activity can take up to 10 minutes at a time, perhaps once or twice a week. One thing I did notice, however was that when I had my hair cut, the grey hair became more noticeable again. This was because the dark hair was now not much longer than the shorter grey hair. So, I needed to spend some time cutting the grey hairs back a bit further after a haircut. So whip out the scissors and get to work if you are perturbed by your hair starting to go grey.

An interesting thing I notice about grey hair is that when it is wet, say just after a shower, then it tends to darken. This is also true if you put a little oil on it; not something I personally do but it could be a useful treatment for greying hair. Of course, it isn't only hair on your head that turns grey – it can happen all over your body, so you might need to keep an eye out and get your scissors employed on other locations too. It could be a shock to discover that an area where you normally shave has become very grey since the last time you saw it! I have heard stories of men going away for a relaxing vacation, so not taking their razor and being horrified that they had started to grow a rather greying beard!

If all else fails of course, a non-natural solution is to colour your hair and most females are quite happy doing this anyway. However, ladies, please avoid the pink or blue rinse – this immediately gives your age away. Also, jet black hair colour may be too stark and could look artificial, so try dark brown instead. Another option is to use one of the products that replaces the melanin. This is the reason the hair goes grey in the first place because the hair follicle is no longer providing the hair shaft with melanin. I have tried out one of these creams and it certainly seems to work. However, it needs to be applied every few days and seems to be under a cloud because it contains lead acetate. As for hair dyes, I have to say that I am rather suspicious of them. The mere thought of them brings to mind several males that I have seen with strangely orange hair. It looks like they have tried to cover their grey hair and something has gone horribly wrong. If anyone is aware of what products cause this, please let me know so that I can put it in the next revision of this book so others can avoid the embarrassment! I have also read the instructions on my wife's hair dye and I have to say that I am particularly put off by phrases such as 'perform a skin test for 48 hours before any application' or 'do not use for eyebrows or eyelashes as this could cause blindness'!! There have been worries about hair dyes since the thirties due to the compounds p-phenylenediamine (PPD) and lead acetate in them. PPD is a suspected mutagen which can trigger changes to your DNA. The darker the dye, the more PPD it is likely to contain. One study concluded that career hairdressers had a far greater risk of developing bladder cancer. Further evidence in 1995, showed them to have a higher incidence of non-Hodgkins lymphoma and cancer of the bone marrow. Another study of women who continually dye their hair found them to be at a higher risk of ovarian cancer. So please use with caution,

Each hair strand grows, rests for a while then sheds. It is then replaced. Over 100 hairs are typically discarded every day. Alopecia (hair loss or thinning) occurs when the natural shedding is not replaced by new hair growth or if hair follicles are damaged. So what causes such hair loss? Well apparently hypertension and poor circulation (particularly in the scalp) are two main reasons. I've already mentioned above some ways to increase the circulation. Another important way is simply to exercise regularly. I say simply because it is simple – all we have to do is just get out and do it. Another benefit is that with hard enough exercise you will also sweat more and that in itself is good for the health of your hair – it opens the pores of your skin and cleans out the follicles ensuring that they are free from impurities. One likely reason for hypertension is the person being overweight so again, exercising regularly (as well as eating sensibly) will help to keep the weight down. One form of hair loss is traction alopecia which occurs if you pull your hair overly tight such as wearing your hair too firmly braided or pulled back for prolonged periods of time; insert curlers too tightly; or twist your hair continuously. This type of hair loss can result in scarring, which could end in permanent follicle damage. Temporary hair loss can also occur, usually starting 2 or 3 months after a shock to the system from severe stress, high fever, surgery, child birth or menopause; or from a medical or nutritional problem like a vitamin or mineral deficiency, hypothyroidism, chemotherapy, or even starting or stopping medication. This type of hair loss is called telogen effluvium or diffuse hair loss. The good news is that it probably won't cause complete baldness although hair might be lost from all over the head. The hair should begin to return to normal about three months after the problem is corrected.

So what happens if all else fails or you have read this book too late and you have already gone bald? Well I guess if you are female, you would have no problems buying a wig but that doesn't seem to be a particularly socially acceptable approach for males. I have to say that the best solution I have seen is to shave the head. This has become quite a fashionable look and certainly makes a man look much younger than a bald pate or creating a 'comb-over'. Just one small word of caution though – do guard against sunburn and potential skin cancer since this part of your anatomy probably hasn't seen the sun before.

Clearly there are some hair styles that will make you look older – this is true for males and females. In fact a bad hair-do can age you more than your face so if you're not sure, spend plenty of time looking through magazines or consulting a good hairdresser. Recall the well known saying – "Life is an endless struggle full of frustrations and challenges, but eventually you find a hair stylist you can trust."! Women probably have much more flexibility in the number and types of hairstyles that they can wear and therefore of looking younger (or older!). Ponytails can appear to take years off most women's faces. In fact, just wearing their hair long and loose can also make them look more youthful.

One intriguing thing you notice about some men with thinning hair is that they decide to grow a moustache as if, somehow to make up for the reduction in overall hair. All I can say is – beware, it seems to be a bit of a giveaway.

Review of Chapter 1

Here are some of the things that you might have taken note of if you want to avoid thinning and to keep your hair in good condition –

- The use and abuse of combs and brushes and how your fingers can help.
- How massaging your scalp can be more beneficial than simply shampooing your hair.
- The dangers of using hairdryers and hair products.
- Why rinsing your hair thoroughly is so important.
- How to tug at your hair to strengthen it.
- The benefits of the head banging exercise.
- Using affirmations and visualisation while doing all these activities.
- The importance of sweating frequently.
- What to do if you are already balding significantly.

Chapter 2 - Your Face and Neck

This is probably the chapter that most people will be interested in because the face is the most visible part of our body, the one that we look at every day and the area where we and others first notice the ravages of time. That fearful cry of 'my God, I have a wrinkle' is often heard in somebody's 30s and from thereon becomes a frequent 'Oh my God, I have another wrinkle'! Well I am continuously being told how few wrinkles I have and frequently asked how I have prevented them. As even Ava Gardner is believed to have said "My face, shall we say, looks lived in."

So this is the chapter you've been waiting for. This is where I explain how to prevent your face getting wrinkled and aged too quickly and even how to rejuvenate those faces that have already succumbed to father time. This section covers a whole range of items from magic potions and makeup to exercises, sunlight, massage and smoking. But perhaps most important of all is the detailed description of Facial Isometric exercises. One thing you will not find is a description or advice about cosmetic surgery. This book is about how to look youthful naturally. There are some pretty horrific stories about such surgery going wrong and some obvious examples of subjects who have clearly gone too far. If you risk ending up looking stretched, misshapen, reworked to excess or unnatural, I personally do not see the point.

Let me say right up front that I rarely use creams and potions on my face (nor on the rest of my skin for that matter). To me, it seems clear that all of these products are a waste of time. Just look at all the people that use them and tell me honestly where's the rejuvenation benefit? It's a well known fact that the majority of the cost of cosmetics (apart from the huge profits) is in marketing and packaging. Even moisturisers I have hardly ever used unless my skin had been particularly affected by drying out in the sun or wind. In fact, if you read the labels on these products then read up on the ingredients, you might be appalled at how potentially dangerous some of these chemicals are. I'm sure many of you know people who have reacted badly to some of them. Some products even warn you to try them on an 'unimportant' skin surface to check! Even more of a worry is the way that many people simply apply several of these products one after the other, effectively using their skin as a chemical laboratory. I have also never had a facial in my life. Not that I wouldn't enjoy having my face massaged but when I realised that the main intention seems to be to rub in as many creams and chemical products as possible in half an hour to an hour then I was not going to put up with that! The same applies to mudpacks. You may not realise it but cosmetics are not regulated by the FDA (Food and Drug Administration in the U.S. and similar bodies in other countries), so skin care products do not have to be proven safe! Now don't misunderstand me; if I had a physical issue that needed a medicinal cream then of course I would use that (such as antiseptic, sunscreen, anti-fungicidal, sting or burn repair …).

Perhaps even more surprising to many of you is that I almost never wash my face with soap (nor for that matter, with any other cleanser, lotion, toner, peeler, etc!). As it happens, I never put aftershave on after shaving either – it always seemed a rather masochistic activity considering all the stinging for no purpose! These may well be further boons for achieving youthful skin. I do however rub my face quite firmly with a towel after washing it, as I do with the rest of my body after a shower. This probably leads to a certain amount of exfoliation which is generally considered good for the skin. Most proponents claim that besides leaving your skin softer and smoother, the friction also boosts your circulation and helps unclog pores. By the way, apparently taking a very hot shower tends to strip the natural oils from the skin which can tend to leave it rather dry. I must say that personally I do not like showering in cool water but on the other hand I cannot take them too hot either.

One subset of the cosmetics industry of course is makeup. Sadly many females (and some males) smother their faces in a variety of colouring and covering agents. As Oscar Wilde apparently wittily phrased it "A woman's face is her work of fiction." At the extreme, in a desperate attempt to improve their looks, some people put on such a cake of makeup that they look worse than if they had left their skin natural. French born actress Claudette Colbert captured it well when she purportedly said "It matters more what's in a woman's face than what's on it." Wearing makeup all the time is also very unfortunate since it prevents the skin ever getting any sunlight. There has been such a lot of publicity about melanoma cancer and how bad UV rays are for your skin that it has all gone overboard. In fact, as in most things, a moderate amount of sunlight is very good for your skin. There is increasing evidence that high levels of vitamin D protect against various cancers particularly those of the digestive system including the mouth and throat. Some vitamin D is present in milk and of course in some multivitamin tablets but the best and natural source is from sunlight triggering your body to produce it. The sun also seems to help your skin produce natural, healthy oils which keep your skin youthful. It is also important to spend at least some time during the day without makeup just to let your poor skin breathe a little! Now I am not suggesting at all that you should spend hours sun baking (sun bathing) but getting 10 – 15 minutes of sunlight (or at least unfiltered daylight) to your skin several days a week will be very beneficial. So even if you live in colder climes where the sun's appearance is infrequent, there are still plenty of beneficial rays on cloudy days. This doesn't mean just your face – you should expose as much of your body as possible. Now we have all seen those weather-beaten folk, often from the country, whose skin has become rather leathery. Rest assured that 10 minutes a day, several times a week will not create that look. In fact this effect is probably caused as much by the wind as by the sun, so I would certainly recommend protecting yourself from the wind. Before receiving complaints from some Bodies, I should make it clear that I certainly do agree with keeping in the shade (outside of the 'medicinal' 10 minutes) or using sunscreen. However, once again, do be aware of the chemicals in sunscreen – I only ever use it if I am going to be directly in the sun. I should add here that there certainly seem to be benefits to wearing sun glasses (good quality ones of course!) while in the sun (especially if you live in a very sunny part of the world like Australia). Not only will they protect your eyes from potential sun damage but they will help avoid squinting which is likely to create wrinkles near your eyes. I refer here not only to actual wrinkles from your muscles starting to permanently tighten but also to apparent wrinkles caused by a suntan that leaves visible lines from those areas not tanned because they have been screwed-up while squinting in the sun.

So what is the 'secret' that I am about to share with you that will definitely keep your face looking more youthful, perhaps 10 or 15 years more youthful?

Well, the main reason that a face (and skin generally) ages is because the multitude of small muscles just under the skin start to sag mainly due to lack of use. In some cases, the issue might be that the muscles have tightened up permanently probably due to stress. Wait a moment, I hear you say, most of my wrinkles are actually 'smile lines' and I still use those muscles to smile. Well that may be true but most muscles in the body have a 'counter' muscle, that is, one that works in the opposite direction. By the way, while it takes 17 muscles to smile, it takes 40 to frown, so just smiling doesn't actually exercise most muscles! In the face, typically, people only use muscles in the one direction (and sadly, many don't even use muscles much in any direction). So the way to overcome this is the very same thing that you would do to prevent other muscles in the rest of your body from atrophying and that is to exercise them. Usually, muscles are attached to bones. However, in the face, most are attached to each other or to the skin and this is why the skin appears to sag when it is actually the muscles sagging. A little known but very important function of our muscles is to act as pumps for the blood and lymph vessels. When the face muscles have lost their normal tone, these fluids are not moved into and out of the facial area and this poor circulation leads to poor complexion and lack of natural, healthy colour. Believe it or not there are 53 muscles in your face and I'm about to explain how I give most of those a workout.

I first came across Facial Isometrics many, many years ago. In fact, back then, isometrics generally was a popular form of exercise and muscle training. Perhaps I should first give an explanation of isometrics. In traditional weight training, weights are used to create opposition to the muscles while they are moved throughout a given range of motion. Isometrics on the other hand has no motion but the muscles are pushing against an immovable object which might indeed be a fixed object or more interestingly other parts of the body, often the same muscle in the opposite side of the body. Having explained this, it is perhaps apparent that so-called "Facial Isometrics" are not actually isometric at all since we will be using the face muscles to move throughout their whole (albeit restricted) range of movement! So perhaps we should look at where and what are the major muscle groups in the face that we are going to work with. Here's a diagram.

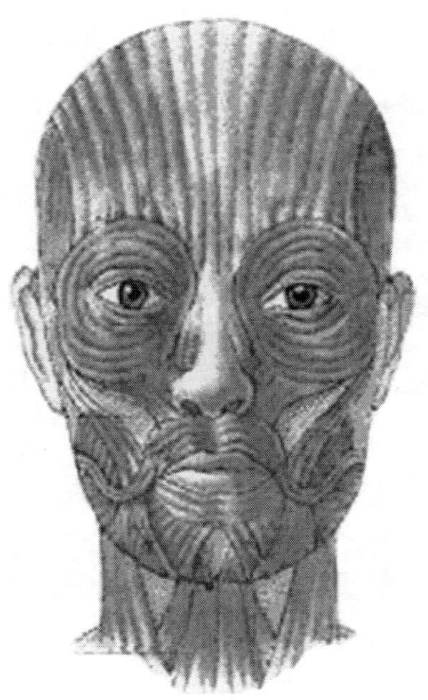

It doesn't look very pretty without the skin does it? But you can see fairly clearly why it is easy to get baggy eyes, loose jowls and so on. You might now also be getting insights into one of the drawbacks to surgical facelifts. These operations simply stretch the skin and cut the excess away but if in addition you do not strengthen the underlying muscles then the new look probably won't last long! Even more disconcerting is the possibility of a poor surgeon removing or stretching muscle by mistake. Another advantage of Facial Isometric Exercises is that they help blood circulation which keeps skin clear, smooth and healthy. I don't see how a face lift can help in these areas. Yet another side benefit is that it releases tension which can really show on your face. With less tension there is also likely to be less headaches. Not something a face lift would cure!

I have been doing these Facial Isometric Exercises for many years. However, don't think that it will take you that long to get results. I believe that you will see positive changes within a few weeks. The whole set of exercises takes me about 10 minutes or so but I do each individual exercise for about 50 repetitions. When you start, you will probably only do about 10 - 20 repetitions (known as reps) and gradually build up. Those of you that have worked out with weights in the gym will know that if you work hard enough you can get a 'burning' sensation in your muscles. Serious muscle builders work hard to achieve this intensity. Since you hardly ever use these face muscles, you will probably experience this burning feeling. I suggest that you don't do more than 2-3 extra reps with this particular muscle after feeling this sensation. I usually vary the speed at which I perform the reps – some I do longer and slower, others I do faster. For reasons that I cannot remember, I usually start by working on the muscles alongside my mouth and working down to my neck then starting again just above my mouth and working up to my forehead. However, to keep things in a simple order, we'll start at the neck and work up. With many of the muscle groups that are replicated on each side of the face, we will be repeating the following pattern – do left side, do right side, alternate left and right, do both sides together. This way you will be really working them out! One other word of advice – when you first start doing these exercises, look at yourself in the mirror to ensure that you really are working the relevant specific muscles. Some of you will be a bit put off by what you are seeing but once you get the hang of it, you can do it anywhere you feel comfortable (which for most people means where nobody can see them!).

So here we go –

1. neck and under chin

a) Tilt your head back to stretch the skin under your chin. To help initially with this exercise, feel the muscle running from your chin down the front of your neck and tense it. You might find this difficult to do at first so tilt your head back, open you mouth and now lift your lower jaw to close your mouth as you tense the muscle. Tense it at least 10 times then do it a few times with your head less tilted. Another way to think of this exercise is to tilt your head backwards while lifting your chin upwards. Hold this position while making chewing motions with your jaw.

b) Now press your chin downwards hard against your neck (or probably the middle of your collar bone) so as to compress the muscle and skin then tilt your head back slightly as you tense the muscle again. Do this at least 10 times.

2. sides of neck

a) The muscles at the side of your neck are larger and probably easier to tense than the one in exercise 1. Again you might like to feel the muscle with your fingertips to help. Tense the left side at least 10 times then swap to the right side. Now alternate left and right 10 times. Then do a set of tensing both sides at the same time. This last one might take some practice!

b) Now repeat the whole thing all over again but this time first press your chin downwards hard against the side of your neck (or probably the side of your collar bone) then tilt your head back slightly as you tense the muscle again. Do this at least 10 times for each movement.

I've seen some people lift up their chin and slap the neck skin with the back of their hand. I've never done this but if you think it might be helpful, you could add that here.

3. sides of chin

a) Now we are going to work on the muscles that run from your bottom lip diagonally down to the bottom of your jaw. This might take some practice so use your fingers and look in the mirror particularly for these. So tense the left side at least 10 times. You will know that you have got it when your lower lip is dragged down and diagonally to the left. Then swap to the right side. Now alternate left and right 10 times. Then do a set of tensing both sides at the same time.

b) Now we are going to use the muscles in the opposite direction. This will also include the muscles of the lower lip in an upwards and diagonal direction. So starting with the left side, you will look as though you have dragged the bottom left of your lower lip up across to your upper lip – not a pretty sight but it will prepare you for a gnurdling competition! Then swap to the right side. Now alternate left and right 10 times. Then do a set of tensing both sides at the same time (this is really quite strange and difficult so work on it).

4. lower lip

We've already worked on the lower lip in an upwards motion in exercise 3. Now we'll counterbalance that by pulling the lower lip downwards. This looks like a pout. To avoid making it too easy by assisting with the upper lip pushing down, open your mouth a bit.

5. sides of mouth

While doing these, make sure that you concentrate on using the muscles all the way out to the edge of your face – don't just use your lip muscles.

a) The action is to pull the side of the lip straight out to the side. As usual, firstly do the left side for at least 10 times, then the right side, then alternate left and right and finally stretch out both sides at the same time.
b) Now to use the opposing muscles, pull the left end of your lip away from your jaw-line and towards the centre of your mouth. Repeat on the right side; alternate; then both sides in together.

To finish off here, alternate the last movements of 5 a) and b), that is, both ends in then both ends out 10 times making sure you complete it with both sides out – I say this because I would rather my mouth 'remembers' to smile out than pucker in! Remember the saying "I've never seen a smiling face that was not beautiful."

6. mouth to ears

This is one of my favourites and is what a basic face lift is trying to accomplish. That is, to lift the jowls and ends of the lips out and up towards the ears.

a) So starting with the left side, pull the corner of your mouth diagonally up towards your ear. Do this at least 10 times where some of them are really pulling so hard that you are pulling your ear down slightly (some of you will find this easier to actually achieve than others but you should at least be getting this feeling). Continue right, alternate, both sides together.

b) Now of course, do the whole thing in the opposite direction. This tends to use the muscle in the upper lip mostly but try to use muscle as far up the cheek as possible. Now I tend to prefer my muscles' memory to be a smile rather than concluding with this strange frown so I finish off by creating a false smile for a count of ten. Alternatively you could do these exercises in reverse (i.e. b before a)

Notice that while doing some of the exercises you will find it easier to isolate the necessary muscles by opening your mouth a bit and even moving your jaw sideways.

7. upper lip and nose

a) So we've worked the sides of the upper lip in a downwards direction in 6 b). So now lift the middle half of your upper lip hard and scrunch it up to your nose ten times.
b) Now lift the left side of your upper lip straight up the side of your nose. Continue right, alternate, both sides together (this last one is a bit hard to distinguish from 7 a) but try to notice the difference using a mirror and your fingertips. To explain the difference, this exercise is concentrating on the lip muscles below and at the side of the nose, whereas 7 a) is working the upper lip muscle directly under the nose.
c) Now for the opposite of 7 a), which consists of pulling the middle of the upper lip downwards past your upper teeth.
d) Finally a much harder movement. This is using muscles at the edges of the lower nose and partially the one immediately above the upper lip. To do this, you must concentrate on keeping the upper lip still and using the small muscles to pull the nose downwards. I always find that I cannot do this for as many reps as other exercises as it tends to burn quickly.

8. around eyes

In addition to loose jowls, the skin around the eyes is probably most responsible for showing the effects of ageing. The two main issues are bagginess and darkness under the eyes, plus crows-feet or wrinkles extending out from the corners of the eyes. There is one point of potential good news here (again I'm afraid that it only seems to apply to men) and that is that many women seem to consider the 'scrunches' at the side of the eyes rather sexy!

Let's start with under the eyes. Some reasons I've heard for causing bagginess and dark rings are poor circulation and build-up of fluids like lymph. Well, for either of these causes, the following will help alleviate it. Just a word of warning – this exercise may leave the area under your eyes looking rather more wrinkled for about ten minutes before the improvement occurs, so do not do it just before going into a meeting or a special rendezvous!

a) Basically, the exercise consists of using the muscles under the eyes to pull the skin up towards the eyes. You will probably need to do it initially in front of a mirror to see it in action and you will see and feel it pulling the top half of your cheek up but it is the muscles directly under the eyes that you should be using not those in the cheek. As normal, do 10 reps on the left side then the right followed by alternating left and right then pulling up both sides together, I find this exercise can be improved even more by firstly pulling down the top lip and lower cheeks (with the corresponding muscles) and holding that position while performing the eye exercise.

Apparently, crow's feet are caused by such things as too much sunbathing, squinting from the sun (which eventually becomes a permanent muscle tension) and smoking. We'll talk about the many evil effects of smoking later but you can help avoid squinting by wearing sunglasses and a hat when in the sun, also by wearing reading glasses if you need them! As previously mentioned, if you are squinting while getting a suntan then you will inevitably end up with white squint lines which cause an effect which looks like crow's feet.

Unfortunately I cannot find any way to use facial muscles to pull the skin out away from the eyes towards the ears, nor down towards the cheeks. However, we can pull it upwards towards the forehead and we will cover this in the forehead exercise below. We can also work the muscles in the same way that crinkles up the side of the eyes in the first place. Why would you want to do something that causes the problem, I hear you asking, Well it is a common way to relax a muscle – to tense it hard then relax it. When the muscle relaxes, it ceases to 'scrunch' up the area. This is how Botox injections work – the toxin paralyses the muscle so it no longer works. But they only last for a while (typically 3 to 8 months) and then the muscle tenses up again when the deadening chemical wears off and the problem returns. With this exercise and other relaxation activities, you can get rid of the underlying cause for good.

b) Use the muscles in your cheek to lift it up hard towards your eyebrow. It is a bit like a squint. As usual do this left, right, alternate, both together but after each set relax for a moment before continuing. At the end of all four sets, relax again then open up your eyes and the area around them as wide as possible for a count of ten. This will relax the cheek muscles back down again.

c) A firm massage of the (potential) crow's feet area will also be beneficial. Simply rub your finger-tips up and down about ten times and then rub them from the corners of your eyes outwards.

9. eyelids

I also exercise the eyelids. While it is not much of a problem for most people, for some there can be a certain build-up of bagginess there. Anyway, I do it for completeness. So, simply blink the eyes shut and open for your requisite number of times, ensuring that for some of them you completely open your eyes wide before closing them again. Then repeat this looking as far down as possible then again looking as far up as possible. If you feel you need more work in this area then you can do the usual left, right, alternate, both routine.

10. forehead

There are many who have permanently furrowed brows. Like crow's feet, this is usually due to permanently tensed muscles. As explained above, we will tense these muscles then relax them. As it happens, the first exercise also stretches the crows feet area upward somewhat, so helps there also.

a) Use the muscles in your forehead to pull upwards then release. This should raise your eyebrows up and furrow your brow. Every so often, hold it up tight before releasing. When you have finished your requisite number of repetitions, close your eyes and relax for a short while then squeeze your eyes tight before opening. By the way, while furrowing up your forehead with this exercise, you could hold it there and do the under eye exercise as an alternative to exercise 8 a). Actually, I usually do both.
b) Now we pull the forehead down the other way, so that the eyebrows move downwards, like a frown then release. This will probably also pull the eyebrows inwards together.
c) Finally, alternately raise and lower the eyebrows. I usually finish with one long pull upwards and open my eyes as wide as possible then add a strong smile as well.

Now this might seem like a lot of exercise time to squeeze into your busy day. But in fact, once you've got the sequence, doing 10 reps takes about 5 seconds or so which means that the whole lot only takes about 6 minutes! Once you increase the repetitions, it will take longer but by then you will have seen the results starting to show and be keen to incorporate it into your normal daily routine. I actually do most of the exercises while driving to or from work so it takes no extra time at all! Just be careful – there are some things you shouldn't do while actually driving but you can do while stopped at traffic lights or when you get to your destination. Alternatively, you could do these exercises while doing the housework, watching TV, or wherever! I do this whole group of exercises once a day as many days a week as possible, so usually 4 – 5 times a week.

As already mentioned, some ageing of the face is due to lack of muscle use and some is due to stress causing the muscles to tense up, usually creating lines and wrinkles, especially around the eyes and forehead. The exercises above will help both situations. The tension related issues can also be alleviated by a variety of stress relief activities and there is a later chapter on this. As I mentioned before, Botox injections are used to numb the poor muscles so that they cannot contract. Goodness knows what this does to the overall condition of the face muscles over time. Of course there are also several side-effects that can occur with Botox injections including headache, neck pain, bruising and nausea. Anyway, it must be much healthier and natural to relieve the tension with massage and other stress relief activities.

So here are some massages that you will find very beneficial to do at least once a week. These are probably best done with your eyes closed.

1. Forehead

a) I release any residual tension by using my finger and thumb of both hands, starting at the inside of my eyebrows and squeezing, working my way up towards my hairline. Then I come down to my eyebrows again but a little further out and work up again, continuing moving outwards to just past the end of my eyebrows. This is good for any furrowed lines you might have.

b) Then for the scrunched up middle of your eyebrows, you need to put the fingertips of both hands in the middle of your eyebrows and gently and slowly pull them across to the ends of your eyebrows. Do this about ten times.

2. Edge of eyes

With the back of your forefingers, rub your temples beside your eyes up and down fairly firmly about ten times. Then holding the backs of your forefinger and middle fingers at the edge of your eyes press and pull them firmly out to your temples. Repeat about ten times.

3. Eyes generally

An excellent way to relax your eyes, especially if you have been doing a lot of reading, computer work or squinting is to do some palming. Rub your palms together fairly fast until they feel warm. Then cup them over your closed eyes and hold for a while as you breathe slowly.

As some folk age, they tend to develop a greyish pallor. This is usually due to poor circulation in the skin. This is improved tremendously by the facial exercises above but also by general body exercise, especially if it makes you sweat somewhat. Another reason men might have that pallor is if they do not shave regularly or properly and have grey stubble!

The neck is an area that particularly shows ageing. The skin starts to get baggy and loose. Some people cover this up by wearing scarves or high collars. Some of the exercises described above are designed specifically to address this issue. A stiff neck is frequently an affliction of older people but it can be avoided or remedied by some simple exercises. Since I believe in preventive actions rather than remedial ones, I recommend you do these exercises several times a week, preferably daily. They are included in the set of daily exercises described in a later chapter but I will explain these neck ones right now. They can be done standing or sitting and should be carried out fairly slowly and gently.

So, holding the shoulders, arms and upper torso still, start by twisting your head gently to the left (and remember what you can see there), now twist it the opposite way to the right (and remember what you can see there). Now repeat to the left but try to see a bit further around. Do the same to the right. Repeat this a total of about ten times. You might hear a slight crunching sound as you twist your neck around – this means you really need this exercise! Do not use your hands to help push your head further than you can naturally twist it as this might cause some damage.

Next, lay your head down to the left so that your left ear comes close to your left shoulder. You probably will not be able to touch your ear on your shoulder but this is fine. Now lay it over to the right side. All the time, keep facing forwards. Repeat this a total of about ten times.

Now, hang your head down forwards so that your chin comes down towards your throat. Again, you might not be able to touch it but that's OK. Lift it back up straight. Repeat this for a total of about ten times.

Finally, hang your head down forwards so that your chin comes down towards your throat again and now roll it from left to right. Do this about ten times. This exercise used to be done by rolling a complete circle around the back but that is now considered to be bad for the vertebrae as it might wear them down. (I will make no comment about that theory!)

One interesting point that I will mention here, is that I never suffer from headaches. I don't know exactly what I can attribute this to but I suspect it is a combination of regular head, neck and scalp massaging and the neck exercises. Frequent meditation (see chapter on Stress Relief) probably also helps.

One final subject I must include in this chapter about the face is the damage done by smoking. The discolouration that smokers develop around the mouth and often right up the face is very ageing, let alone an indication of the damage done. It is particularly revolting when it affects the teeth and moustache. Of course, smoke is especially damaging to the eyes and not only is fading eyesight not going to help present a youthful appearance but nor is the opaque colouring the smoker's eyes often develop. One other thing I've noticed about smokers is that their lips become very wrinkled up and old looking. I can only assume that this is due to the constant puckering of the lips holding cigarettes in them. I hope that some of the Facial Isometric exercises above will help here but I have no idea since I have never smoked. Smokers, email me and let me know how much they help and also seriously consider finding a way to quit.

I thought that I had said enough about the cosmetics industry and sufficiently mentioned my concerns about overuse and the potential dangers of the chemicals involved. However, I have just noticed an article in a newspaper and if even only half of what was written is true, I feel obliged to pass on the information, which was mainly addressing some of the moral and ethical implications. One case cited was a cosmetics company which used the skin from executed Chinese criminals to create an ingredient for their lip and anti-wrinkle products. The assumption was that having done a deal with the prison authorities, their products were produced more cheaply than other companies using human skin from other sources. Some of these sources by the way, for procedures such as lip implants also come from corpses (even from countries such as the U.S.A.). These are most often victims of car accidents where the bereaved relatives are convinced to sign consent forms, presumably assuming their loved one's bodies will help genuine humanitarian uses! Here's another gruesome one – It appears that there's an anti ageing, anti wrinkle cream on the market where the active ingredient is derived from the foreskin of a circumcised baby! In addition, the article mentioned the name of a clinic in Moscow attended by many foreigners where so-called anti-ageing injections consist of cells from umbilical cords and placentas of aborted foetuses. There is also a selection of shampoos and face masks from placentas! I can only assume that similar clinics exist elsewhere too. All far too gory for me to contemplate very much but each to their own!! Users of these products often don't care or would rather not ask about the ingredients in items they are using but if you have any moral compunction, I suggest you research a bit yourself. I have the names of some of these products and services but decided not to reveal them in this book.

Review of Chapter 2

Suggestions in this chapter for helping you attain a youthful looking face included –

- Consider the dangers of using too many chemicals on your face. Moreover re-evaluate whether these magic potions are actually benefiting you. Even cleansers, soaps and aftershave are suspect.
- Facials might be pleasant but are they achieving anything and are they just an excuse to use your face to mix a cocktail of expensive chemicals? Similar questions might be asked about mudpacks.
- The pros and cons of sunlight and wind.
- Carry out the facial isometrics many days per week.
- How to massage your face regularly.
- Help avoid a stiff neck by performing the specific exercises.
- Quit smoking.

Chapter 3 - Glasses and your Eyesight

Apart from lines and crows feet discussed in the previous chapter, there are two main topics to discuss with regards to the eyes and how they affect how old you look. The first of course is tired and worn-out looking eyes (although this can affect anybody at any age!) and the other is the fact that from the age of 40, most people's eyesight starts to deteriorate. So we will look at subjects such as sleep, lighting, special exercises, food, hydration, disease and glasses.

The most common age-related problem with eyesight is that the lenses of the eyes toughen and lose their elasticity over time and eventually for many of us this causes problems with short range vision. This is called presbyopia. It is different from 'straightforward' short-sightedness, or myopia. You certainly feel like you are ageing when you have to start taking out your glasses to read and many people look older when they are wearing glasses. It is worth noting that if you have never had any eyesight problems until presbyopia then you probably do not actually need prescription glasses. You will almost certainly want to go to a professional optician at first but when you realise that the $10 spectacles containing magnifying lenses in a supermarket or gas (petrol) station work just as well then you might do as I do – I have a pair of prescription spectacles but I also have lots of the significantly cheaper ones lying around at home, in the car and at work.

I can still remember the feeling, the first time I realised that I could no longer see up close – I was putting my head into a cupboard to tighten the screws on the door hinge. I just could not see the screw-head enough to get the screwdriver in. A year or so later, I started to find myself standing up to be able to read the papers on my desk! I also had to hold business cards out at arms length to be able to read them! I clearly had to do something, so I started reading as much as I could about the subject. I came across some eye exercises that certainly helped for a while but I have to admit that it was only a matter of time before I eventually had to resort to wearing glasses. There are some writers that claim that if you perform the exercises then you will not need glasses at all but I personally couldn't keep them at bay for more than a few years. I am amazed that somebody hasn't yet discovered a way to soften the eye lens, they would make a fortune!

I will describe here some of the exercises that I found useful. Generally, they are designed to strengthen the muscles that stretch or shorten the lens but eventually the lens seems to get too tough for the muscles to be able to function enough. The other important fact is that it is not only the lens that focuses the light – the cornea plays an even more important role and that is not helped much by muscle exercises. It would seem sensible therefore to protect your corneas from the ravages of the elements, particularly sun and wind; and most definitely from smoke!
The Palming & Blinking exercises already mentioned in the Facial Isometrics section are useful here but more specific are the following –

a) Look as far left as possible without moving your head then as far right as possible. Repeat back and forth about ten times. Now look up as far as possible, then down and repeat ten times. Do the same thing looking diagonally up left and down diagonally right. Also do it looking diagonally up right and down diagonally left. Then circle your eyes around clockwise pushing your vision out as far as possible and also do it in reverse anticlockwise.

b) Hold your thumb upright and touch it to your nose. Focus on the lines of the knuckle. This will probably be hard to do and cause a slight muscle 'burn'. Move your thumb out slowly as far as your arm will allow, focussing hard all the way. Bring it back in and out several times keeping your focus on the knuckle. Now bring it in to about 3 inches (7 cms) away and focus on the knuckle then focus out to an object in the distance. Repeat back and forth about ten times. Now move the thumb out to about 5 inches (12 cms) and focus on the knuckle then focus in hard to the tip of your nose (again this might be difficult and cause a slight muscle burning sensation). Repeat back and forth about ten times. Some of the refocussing should be done slowly and some quite rapidly.

I used to do these exercises every morning and sometimes again during the day. It only takes a couple of minutes. I must confess, now that I definitely have to wear glasses to read, I am tending to do them less frequently. However, they are very useful if you get eyestrain – I often use them if I've been reading or working at the computer for too long. By the way, those who have difficulty waking up and getting out of bed in the mornings might find the exercises above a useful way to get the eyes and brain 'in gear'!

Palming is an activity that I do still perform frequently, so I will describe it further here. It was originally a yoga technique but has since been taken up by various 'natural' vision systems. The intention is to calm the visual system. Normally, if no light were entering the eyes, you would see nothing. However, if you have eyestrain, you might see swirling patches of colours. By placing your palms over your eyes, the warmth from the hands helps relax the tense eyeballs and muscles.

So that's what you do – Get into a comfortable position, close your eyes, rub your hands together and place your palms over your closed eyes. Slightly cup your palms so as not to press on the eyeballs but ensure that as much light as possible is blocked out. Allow the warmth of your hands to diffuse gently into your eyes. You can add to this by imagining a peaceful scene. Most importantly, relax. This is a wonderful method of relieving tired, tense, overworked eyes. In turn, those of you who suffer from headaches might also find that this reduces the tension.

You frequently read about Laser Correction operations that can apparently repair your vision. These procedures seem to work pretty well for standard myopia but their solution to presbyopia is novel – they cause one eye to be short sighted and the other to be long sighted (preferably by operating on just a single eye). It then relies on the brain to make some serious readjustments which not everybody's brains can do. When I asked questions about this approach, I never received a satisfactory response as to what happens to your 3-D or stereoscopic vision. I would be intrigued to hear from people who have had laser correction for presbyopia.

Another reason that older people have problems seeing is that they need more lighting to see, particularly in order to read. The size of the pupil governs the amount of light that gets into the eye to eventually reach the retina. The amount that the pupil dilates decreases with age. By the age of 60, your pupils decrease to about one-third of the size they were when you were 20, so older eyes let in much less light. Also, the lens becomes less transparent so less light passes through. I really started noticing how dim it was in hotel rooms and restaurants – mood lighting is one thing but it's a disaster when you cannot read the menu, even with your reading glasses on! So the answer is to have some really good lighting where you want to read. Aim to sit where the best lighting is located. Easier said than done when you are not in your own home! I find that if the lighting is excellent then my vision is frequently good enough to read without my reading glasses.

There is a disease that I should mention here because apparently it is already affecting millions of people around the world. Macular degeneration is a progressive eye condition which attacks the macula of the eye – this is where central vision occurs. Although it rarely results in total blindness, it can leave people with only dim images at the centre of their vision and affect their colour perception. Peripheral vision may not be affected. AMD is Age-related Macular Degeneration. This can destroy the central vision necessary for such activities as driving, reading and other detailed work. There seems to be no medical cure for AMD but the following food advice might be useful -

- Carrots and other orange vegetables are rich in beta-carotene, which apparently protects against age-related macular degeneration (AMD).

- Cold-water fish such as tuna and salmon are believed to improve vision because they contain DocosaHexaenoic Acid (DHA), which is concentrated in the retina and provides structural support to cell membranes. Apparently, regular fish eaters have a 50 per cent lower risk of AMD.

So what if you've been doing your exercises diligently, you've got bright lighting everywhere but there are still times when you have to wear glasses? What should you look out for (no pun intended) in order to avoid looking older? Well first of all, be careful about buying old-fashioned styled frames. Of course the glasses need to be functional but style and fashion in all areas, including your glasses, are clear indicators of age. Bring along a younger friend or family member when choosing the frames or get advice from one of the younger assistants. One particular style to be wary of is bifocals, at least avoid those that have a noticeable, solid line across the middle of the lenses – they are definitely considered to be the glasses of choice for old people! One thing you should avoid doing which is typical of older people who have presbyopia is looking over the top of your glasses at far away objects – simply remove your glasses to look.

And what can be done about those tired old looking eyes? What causes the bags and dark rings? Frequently cited reasons are dehydration, poor circulation and build-up of lymph. The facial isometrics (which you will now already be doing regularly) will certainly help if the cause is bad circulation or fluid retention.

But what about dehydration? Well you know my views on moisturisers and the like – I have never used them and hold no faith in their restorative properties (even when the words are written in French!). I am also intrigued by the fairly recent fad that everybody needs to be continuously consuming copious quantities of water. There seems to be no research at all that has been done to justify the 'eight glasses a day, or else...' philosophy. Would I be too cynical to suggest that it is simply PR by the bottled water companies, especially now that so many of them seem to be owned by large American corporations? Their product sales seem to have skyrocketed over the last decade or so! Annual sales globally are estimated to be as much as ten billion US dollars! I personally do not drink much water at all apart from what I get naturally from fruit and other foods. I would challenge any comparison between my skin and that of over–consumers of water. In fact, as far as your skin is concerned, the outermost layer is composed of dead cells, so I don't see how it can absorb water from within. Hydration of your skin is far more likely to be influenced by external factors such as air temperature and humidity.

Here are some other myths I'd like to refute –

"An hour of sleep before midnight is worth two after midnight". I think this is utter bunkum. Your body has little concern for where midnight is. In fact with daylight saving time and jet travel, midnight changes constantly! Your best sleeping time is predicated on you circadian rhythm and since for most people your internal circadian oscillation is based on a period that is closer to 25 hours than to 24 hours, bed-time will gradually move over a period of time! I hardly ever go to bed before midnight and I never have. I've never noticed that to be a cause of dark rings or bags under my eyes.

"You must have regular sleeping hours". Again, I have never followed this. I go to bed when I am ready and I get up when I need to. Many soothsayers insist that you cannot catch-up on lost sleep. Personal experience tells me this is nonsense. If I do not feel that I have had enough sleep during the (working) week then I will catch-up at the weekend (or while flying on an aeroplane, or whenever). I often nap but usually for less than an hour. To be honest, the only time that I have noticed that I get dark rings under my eyes is when I spend too long in bed, particularly if it is due to my sleep being disrupted or disturbed.

If dark rings are a perpetual problem for you and nothing seems to have worked, try getting a slight tan. This tends to mask the darkness under the eyes somewhat!

There are certain foods which seem to be useful for improving your sight. According to studies reviewed by the U.S. National Eye Institute, some of these are –

- Fish like sardines, salmon, cod, mackerel and tuna. These cold water fish are an excellent source of DHA (DocosaHexaenoic Acid) and Omega 3 oils which could help with dry eyes and improving sight.
- Green leafy vegetables including spinach and kale; also broccoli, corn, green peas and zucchini (a.k.a. courgette). These are rich in carotenoids, especially zeaxanthin and lutein. Lutein is a yellow pigment and helps protect the macula from sun damage. Studies indicate that diets high in lutein and zeaxanthin were likely to reduce the incidence of cataracts. Also research performed at Schepens Eye Research Institute and Department of Ophthalmology, Harvard Medical School concluded that dietary zeaxanthin assists in protecting the retina from light damage.
- Eggs, which contain, sulphur and lutein (in the yolk). Sulphur compounds seem to protect the lens from cataract formation.
- Garlic and onions are also rich in sulphur.
- Red tomatoes and capsicum provide vitamin C, which is linked with lowered cataract risk.
- Blueberries, bilberries and grapes all contain anthocyanosides, which have been claimed to improve night vision. Studies have shown that eating blueberries has resulted in the reduction of eye fatigue. There is an urban myth that bilberries (a.k.a. Creeping Blueberry) were used during the war by British pilots to improve their night vision.
- Apricots are rich in nutrients such as beta carotene and lycopene that help promote good vision.

Once again I have to mention the perils of smoking, this time, with respect to your eyes. Due to the overwhelming evidence which showed a strong association between smoking and eventual blindness, the British Royal National Institute of the Blind launched a serious public education campaign in 2005 to warn the millions of smokers in the U.K. about these dangers to their eyesight. In the U.S., the General Surgeon's Report of 2004 stated that if you smoke, you have a two to three times greater risk of developing cataracts than a non-smoker. According to a review of studies by the Department of Ophthalmology and Visual Sciences at the Chinese University of Hong Kong, there are strong links between smoking and a number of common eye diseases. These include Graves' ophthalmopathy, age-related macular degeneration (AMD), glaucoma and cataracts. The main reason seems to be that cigarette smoke enhances the generation of free radicals and decreases the levels of antioxidants in the blood circulation, aqueous humour, and ocular tissue. Another general effect is a decrease in the blood supply to the eyes. And don't forget the effects of passive smoking including immediate eye irritation.

Review of Chapter 3

In this chapter we looked at –

- Presbyopia and some exercises to improve the situation.

- The effect of lighting.

- Easing eyestrain.

- Styles of eyewear.

- The effects (or otherwise) of sleep.

- Age-related Macular Degeneration.

- Foods that might assist.

- Improving the appearance of tired looking eyes.

- The perils of smoking.

Chapter 4 - Your Nose, Ears and Hearing

This chapter will consider the ageing effects associated with the nose and ears such as hair as well as investigate what are the impediments to hearing ability and are there some myths here? In particular, should you be sticking something in your ear? Certainly preventative actions will be addressed since there seems to be little that can be done to repair damaged hearing apart from physical hearing aids of course. The condition known as rosacea will also be touched on.

There's one certain way for your ears (and your nose as well) to make you look older and that's to allow a crop of hair to grow from them! I've heard it said that it's God's practical joke to take hair from your head and put it on your nose and ears! It is not entirely clear what makes it happen, but one theory is that as you age, the hair follicles in your nose and ears are more affected by the hormone testosterone, which stimulates the unwanted hair growth. Since the levels of oestrogen in females diminish with age then they are also affected by this extra growth of ear and nose hair as well as general face hair. So the answer is clear – trim it! There are dozens of special devices for doing this but I've never bothered with anything more than a pair of small scissors although I also frequently run my electric razor around my nostrils when shaving. I've always considered it to be too painful to pluck hair from the nostrils but it seems to be the best and longer lasting approach for the ears – either with tweezers or simply your finger and thumb nails.

In addition to hair growth, there is another condition that tends to occur on and around the nose with age and that is rosacea. This disorder is characterized by redness, pimples, and in advanced stages, thickened skin not only around the nose but even extending to the cheeks and eyes. Interestingly it is more common in women, particularly during menopause although the popular picture is of an overweight port-drinking male! However a condition called rhinophyma also may develop in some men although it is rare in women. This is characterized by an overgrown, bulbous, red nose which is caused by an enlargement of the sebaceous glands beneath the surface of the skin. Apparently, rosacea cannot be cured and it rarely reverses itself, although I'm certain that I know of at least one case where antibiotics cleared it up. It would seem that only help from a dermatologist can successfully control and hopefully improve the effects of rosacea. Some natural activities that can help are reducing and managing stress and avoiding over-long periods in the sun. Too much sun exposure heats the skin, which dilates capillaries and can lead to flushing. Of course the other thing to avoid is excessive alcohol (apparently fortified wine like port and sherry is worst) since it dilates the blood vessels and often induces flare-ups in people prone to rosacea.

Your hearing tends to deteriorate as you age and this brings to mind the classic cartoon of an old codger with a hearing horn. If you are middle-aged (does that really still mean somebody over 40?) then having a visible hearing aid certainly gives the impression of you looking older still. However, we should take to heart these words from a U.S. hearing expert "An untreated hearing loss is more noticeable than hearing instruments." Nowadays, of course there are several companies supplying very small hearing aids which can hardly be seen, so if you have serious hearing problems then you can easily locate one of these device suppliers through a health professional. Presbycusis is the term for hearing loss due to age. It is not a single disease, rather a category for the cumulative effects of aging on ones hearing, although it certainly does not affect everybody. Typically hearing loss of this type doesn't start until about 60 years of age. It tends to affect men more than women and usually results in difficulty hearing high-pitched tones. So it is true that older men find it hard to hear a woman's voice! There seems to be no known cure apart from amplification with hearing aids. Cochlear implants are only suitable for very serious loss of hearing.

The Australian Government have a programme of free hearing tests for the over 55s. Well at age 57, I actually received a phone enquiry from them and I decided to partake of the service. I was very pleased to find that my hearing was above average in every respect. I was a little surprised considering that I have always ignored some traditional words of wisdom. I have frequently attended loud rock concerts and discotheques and always turned the music up loud at home! However, perhaps I have not subjected my ears to as much or to such loud noises as some others. All experts seem to agree that loud sounds can injure delicate parts of the ear but it can often be avoided by wearing protection such as earplugs. I've just returned from the Australian Formula One Grand Prix where I had a taste of the discomfort caused by extremely loud noise and I must confess that I and most other spectators were wearing earplugs! Apparently noise induced hearing loss is the most common cause of hearing issues among American adults. It can be due to a single loud sound, such as an explosion or long-term exposure to such sounds as rock music or workplace noise. Even recreational activities could be responsible such as a loud engine in a lawnmower, car or boat.

One piece of advice I have certainly ignored is not to put anything in your ear – I believe that it is important to ensure that your ears are properly dried after a shower or swimming. I see many people who do not bother and wonder about the health of their ears – I have never had an ear infection, trouble with ear wax, or any other such problem. I dry my ears by taking a corner of the towel and twisting it gently into my ear. Perhaps this is another reason why my hearing is still so good. However, I am certainly not suggesting that it is OK to stick thin, pointed or sharp objects into your ears!

If you are already having any hearing problems, here's some things you might do to make it less obvious. Make sure you can clearly see the person speaking. Face them and ensure their face is not in shadow. If you can see the body language and other visual clues then you might be able to fill-in some of the blanks where you don't hear properly. If you have severe hearing problems then you will be very sympathetic to this statement by Ludwig Van Beethoven who apparently said - "Oh you men who think or say that I am malevolent, stubborn, or misanthropic, how greatly do you wrong me. You do not know the secret cause which makes me seem that way to you. Oh how harshly was I flung back by the doubly sad experience of my bad hearing."

I have always been cautious about some of the more outrageous claims made for aromatherapy although you have probably noticed that certain smells can undoubtedly have various effects on the brain. However, here is a study which was presented by reputable psychologists and is very relevant to age. For some strange reason, they studied the possible effects of three aromas on a person's age perception. It seems that grape and cucumber were of no consequence but grapefruit did the trick for men! The male observers assessed the ages of females in photos as several years younger while smelling grapefruit aroma. For female participants it made little difference whether there was any fragrance or none at all. It's unclear whether this outcome is due to a relaxation response or sexual arousal or what but ladies, forget all those expensive perfumes and slap on the grapefruit juice!!

Review of Chapter 4

This chapter looked at the ageing effect of hair in and around the ears and nose and the simple solution for it. Some possible causes of hearing losses were reviewed together with avoidance tactics. The conventional wisdom of not sticking anything in the ears was questioned. Presbycusis was touched on and the subject of hearing aids considered. There were also some suggestions on making any hearing loss less obvious. The age-old condition of rosacea was investigated and some proposals were made for helping reduce its effects or at least to avoid worsening it.

Chapter 5 - Your Teeth

I guess you can have bad looking teeth at any age but there's nothing more suggestive of old age than having to wear dentures. In this chapter you might find some novel approaches and personal views on the activities of brushing teeth, eating sweets and candies, massaging gums and smoking but perhaps you will consider as controversial my opinions on dentists, flossing and other subjects.

Caring for your teeth starts in childhood with good eating habits. I never ate sweets (or candies or lollies) as a child and I'm sure that set a good foundation for healthy teeth. I also rarely indulge as an adult. So if you have the bad habit of snacking on them, I suggest you consider stopping and replacing them with something less harmful to your teeth. Nor did I drink so called 'soft drinks' – a euphemism for 'sugar-loaded' and I have seldom drunk them as an adult either. The contents of soft drinks (a.k.a. soda) include sugars such as corn syrup, acid, dye, and in many, also caffeine. An average can contains about ten teaspoons of sugar plus carbonic or phosphoric acid. Now the sugar in these drinks is bad enough and will cause tooth decay and obesity; however the acid is the hidden danger here! The acid dissolves the calcium out of tooth enamel leaving them softened so bacteria can cause severe damage. So even drinking low-sugar products is not safe for your teeth. Recent research at the University of Maryland Baltimore Dental School shows that soft drinks, especially light-coloured drinks, and including canned iced tea appear to "aggressively" attack teeth. Surprisingly, non-cola varieties caused far more damage than darker drinks. The colas contain phosphoric and citric acids which were shown to be harmful to enamel. The non-cola ones contain malic acid and other organic acids which are even more corrosive to teeth. Also other studies have indicated that phosphorus in cola can make calcium less available. Additionally kidneys in the over forty age group are less able to excrete excess phosphorus making the situation worse. So, in summary, tooth decay and loss, periodontal disease, and gingivitis can result from consuming too many soft drinks.

Another important point is whether you are cleaning your teeth correctly. It is surprising how many people do not seem to be brushing properly. I don't know if this is taught in schools today but I doubt it and it certainly wasn't when I was at school. I must say it came as quite a surprise to me in my teens when I read that you don't just brush from side to side and most of the population only do this on the front facing side of the teeth! So in case you don't know, here's a quick lesson on how to brush your teeth correctly! The basic principle is, instead of brushing across your teeth, you should brush from the gums down the teeth and you do this for each and every tooth. So starting, say, at the left side, upper set at the back on the outside of the teeth, put the toothbrush on the gum and brush down to the end of the tooth and repeat so that the brush lifts up and then moves down from gum to tooth a few times. Move across to the next tooth and repeat the action. Do this for every tooth until you reach the last one on the right then move to the rightmost lower set at the back and repeat across to the leftmost. Now do the same for the inside of the teeth. You should also ensure that you brush between the teeth, not just the outer edges. You can finish off by brushing along the top of your teeth; upper set and lower set with particular emphasis on those right at the back (The wisdoms, if your dentist hasn't pulled them out 'just in case'). This whole activity takes time, probably a few minutes, so don't rush it by missing any teeth.

More recently, I've also taken to brushing my tongue but this is more to ensure my breath remains fresh since it apparently removes the bacteria that cause bad breath. My conclusion is that massaging the gums is far more important than brushing the teeth. Most teeth problems are caused by gum disease, so this is where you should concentrate during your apparent tooth cleaning activity. In fact after cleaning my teeth, I always spend some time specifically massaging my gums with the toothbrush. There is apparently a lot of evidence that germs from gum disease can also cause heart disease!

Conventional wisdom suggests using a soft brush – I have always used at least a medium! Certainly, replacing it every 3 months or so seems appropriate. However, we are also recommended to clean our teeth at least twice a day and to floss as well. I have to say that I have hardly ever cleaned my teeth more than once a day. It's not uncommon to clean teeth before going out to a function to freshen the mouth but there are many other ways to achieve sweet smelling breath apart from using toothpaste. The literature is full of recommendations to brush at least twice a day but none of it seems to be accompanied by any evidence to prove that that is necessary to keep your gums and teeth healthy; in fact it is just as likely that over-brushing could cause damage. One particular concern that has reached my attention of late is the use of dubious chemicals in tooth-pastes. The following warning quote from the packets of popular brands of toothpaste in the U.S.A. should certainly cause us concern about how frequently we decide to put these products in our mouths – "Keep out of the reach of children under 6 years of age." and "If you accidentally swallow more than used for brushing, seek professional help or contact a poison control center immediately". Now I believe this relates mainly to the potential dangers of ingesting too much fluoride but there are two other ingredients found in most toothpastes which also pose health risks if too much is ingested, according to a company in the industry. One is sorbitol and the other is sodium lauryl sulphate. One of the multitude of different types of toothpaste available is the whitening variety. It may well work but I would caution about using it for long periods, after all it is basically a scouring agent which will eventually take the surface right off of your teeth. While on the subject of the multiple assortment of toothpastes all with their different claims of special capabilities, I am reminded of basic economics theories of monopolistic practices. Most of these dozens of products are all owned by only two or three corporations successfully working on the age old marketing principles to keep out competitors. I have to say that I have never been tempted by such promotion and still use the exact same toothpaste that I have always used!

Also I never floss. I did start flossing once on advice from a dentist but I concluded that it was doing me more harm than good. It seemed to be cutting my gums causing them to bleed and the problem here is that you can expose the root of the tooth and by doing that, you can have issues with the nerve. Also I was not happy about having to force the floss in between my teeth which moved the teeth slightly. This didn't sound like a remedy for healthy teeth nor did the prospect of having lumps of dental floss caught between my teeth! Considering that most Americans did not even brush their teeth until after WW2 (when the returning soldiers had picked up the habit), it is astonishing the huge amount of U.S. based propaganda there is about flossing. I hate to sound cynical but take a look at the floss market - there are strings, tapes, flavoured, waxed, un-waxed, and all kinds of strange flosses. Some of them even have sweeteners. Could it be that, just like the rest of the cosmetics industry, companies are creating huge amounts of PR, shonky institutes and research programmes? Even the mouthwash manufacturers are getting on the bandwagon with research sponsored by them apparently showing that using their product is as good as flossing!

So how frequently should you go to the dentist? Well I am going to be rather controversial here and suggest that one reason I have good teeth is that I hardly ever go to one! The only dental issues that I have had were created years ago when I was at junior (primary) school when it seemed to be considered necessary to pull out or fill teeth for the sake of it. I cannot believe that the one tooth that I had pulled and the two that I had filled could possibly have needed this when they were less than ten years old! In fact at that age, the growth of my teeth would not even have been complete (especially the crowns and roots). I have never had to have any other teeth worked on since then (apart from a filled one needing to be re-worked)! Unfortunately, I was too young at the time to know better or to object to it. I suppose it isn't surprising to me that those persons that frequently go to dentists seem to have the most work done, continuously, on their teeth. What really put me on my guard with the dental profession was when I was

17 and having trouble with my upper inside gum – my lower teeth seemed to be touching it and irritating it, causing some inflammation. I went to a dentist recommended by my friends – apparently he had a very plush surgery. Well I soon found out why. He mentioned the possibility of having a special plate made but better still he proposed that I had a block of gold crowning my back teeth in order to keep my mouth slightly open!! I'm glad to say that I couldn't afford it but even more interesting is that a few years later when I was having a checkup with a different dentist, I mentioned it and his recommendation was that I massage the gum regularly. I have been doing this almost every day since and guess what - I have hardly ever had the problem again.

Since then, I started going for a second opinion whenever a dentist has suggested work be done and sad to say, in every instance the second dentist has either found nothing or more amazingly, recommended work on a totally different tooth! So you can understand why I think you should consider being cautious about rushing off to dentists if you want healthy teeth! Now I'm not implying that you shouldn't get a clean occasionally (though beware of further work, especially not that same day) and certainly you would need attention for something serious like a damaged tooth or severe pain. U.S. comedian Rodney Dangerfield seemed to be showing a different type of scepticism when he allegedly quipped "I told my dentist my teeth are going yellow. He told me to wear a brown tie."

There is a lot of contention that drinking milk helps create healthy teeth because of the calcium in it. At first thought, I was suspicious of this since I have never liked milk and never drank it. However, on reflection, in the English school system, all primary school children (age 5 to 11) were obliged to drink a third of a pint bottle every school-day and in those days you were forced to drink it whether you liked it or not! So perhaps during the period of my teeth development, milk calcium did play a part. In addition, phosphorous, fluoride, and vitamins A, C and D are also important during the formation of teeth especially from conception right up to age 20 and beyond.

Once again, I have to mention smoking. It seems that smokers are four times more likely than non-smokers to have periodontal disease. Apparently, smoking limits the growth of blood vessels which slows down the healing of any damaged gum tissue. Also nicotine causes the blood vessels to contract thus depriving the teeth roots of nutrition. Not to mention the unsightly staining of teeth and tongue caused by tobacco. The famous escapologist Harry Houdini obviously had one of the keys to strong teeth but also had habits as dangerous as smoking if you consider this pronouncement attributed to him "No performer should attempt to bite off red-hot iron unless he has a good set of teeth."!

Review of Chapter 5

Perhaps you found some rather different views on dentists and flossing in this chapter. I also voiced my opinions about type of toothbrush and frequency of brushing. My views on sweets, candies and lollies would have come as no surprise but many of you might have found new information about soft drinks, as well as the best approach to cleaning your teeth. There were various discussions about the importance of protecting your gums. Of course several problems affecting gums and teeth caused by smoking were noted.

Chapter 6 - Your Posture and Lower Back

In this section, we will review some of the ways that posture can make us look older and how to address it. In particular, we will consider back problems and how you can avoid them or if you are already a sufferer then how to help relieve it. This will involve investigating the way we move, various exercises and what health practitioners you might approach (or perhaps avoid) for help.

Apparently, eight out of ten in the population experience back pain sometime in their lives. The more you allow it to take hold, the worse it gets and the more it makes you look old and incapacitated. Lumbago is the term used to describe general lower back pain, although it doesn't seem to be commonly used nowadays. Around the age of forty, I was starting to feel a few back twinges and decided I needed to cure them and to prevent them from causing me any future serious complications. Despite knowing the statistics, I am still amazed at how many suffer needlessly from bad backs. I have done my share of gardening, shifting, carrying, digging, and even, in my fifties, lifting my dance partner; but since following a few simple strategies I have never had any real back problems. The fact is, although painful and incapacitating, most lower-back complaints are not caused by serious medical conditions. They are usually the result of poor muscle tone and improper movement, especially when lifting but also while carrying out some of the most simple and basic of activities.

One simple thing I changed was the way I slept in bed. Instead of sleeping on my front, as I then did, I started sleeping on my side, in a sort of 'foetal' position. This took a while to get used to but after a short time it became quite natural and it certainly helped prevent some of the twinges I had started to feel. Conversely, some sleep on their backs, which can also cause pain in the lumbar region. It also increases the chance of you snoring! So practice sleeping on your side. Of course, one common reason for you getting a bad back is simply that your bed is unsuitable in some way; whether it's too soft, too hard, lumpy or just plain old! It also seems that staying in bed for over-long periods can cause a sore back.

Sitting is another basic function that many of us perform very badly. We are frequently either slouched or twisted or using poor body mechanics in some way. It's interesting how many people think that watching television is a form of relaxation for them, when in fact they are tensing and stressing their bodies in all sorts of bizarre ways – draped over couches, partly on the arms, one leg up, looking sideways at the box and they do this for hours on end! And this is after spending most of the day sitting poorly in an office chair! Most of us know what we should do – most of our mothers told us! Push the backside firmly into the back of the chair and sit up straight! Now this is certainly better than slumping in a chair and will reduce your likelihood of getting bad backaches but I believe that there is a further thing that can improve your chances even more and that is to have the chair back slanted slightly back rather than bolt upright. This will give a lot more support to the back rather than all the weight being supported by the spine itself, which happens when you are completely upright. If you spend a fair amount of time sitting at the computer at home then it is essential to spend sufficient money on a good comfortable chair. It goes without saying that if your work involves a lot of sitting then the responsibility for the purchase should lie with your company though I have known many cases where the employee has been able to influence the decision on exactly which type of chair to get.

Some of the real back-killers are basic activities that we carry out faultily every day. In particular there are the simple acts of shaving for men and putting on make-up for women. Unfortunately most of you undoubtedly do these leaning over a sink or dressing table with your knees straight. Usually, you don't even notice at the time the enormous strain being put on the lower back but over a period it builds up and you soon start to feel it later in the day. The good news is that it is very easy to prevent. If you use a mirror on a dressing table, make sure that there is a knee-hole and sit on a stool pushed well in. If your dressing table does not have a knee-hole then get rid of it or remove the mirror so that you stop using it! If you use a mirror over a sink then again get rid of it! If that's totally out of the question then here's what I started doing years ago – open your feet well apart and bend your knees. This immediately removes the strain. It's hard to get used to it at first but it really works and I've never had back-ache. The other, even simpler solution is to put up a mirror on a blank wall and shave or put on your make-up there. Frequently, I shave with an electric razor in front of the full-length mirror in the bedroom (with nothing between me and the wall it is on). Other activities where you probably lean over things and cause back strain are bed-making and washing up. Again, the back problems can be alleviated by bending the knees. If you've been snow skiing in Europe, you are probably already repeating "Bend ze knees!"

More serious damage is caused to the spine (especially the discs) by improper lifting and pulling movements. The legs have quite large and strong muscles and these should be brought into play rather than just the back muscles. Especially when you lift a heavy object, bend your hips and knees, keeping your back perpendicular before straightening your legs to do the lifting. Anything heavier than 10kgs (or

20 pounds) is probably too heavy for many individuals anyway! The other important thing is to keep the object close to your body – the further away it is, the more the lever effect makes it feel heavier and the more it strains the back. The other golden rule is to never lift and twist at the same time. Always lift first then turn your whole body (moving your feet) to where you are going to put the weight down. By the way, it is not only lifting but also putting the object back down when these points should be observed. Most of us are aware of these basic rules but many seem to ignore them at their peril – make it a habit to incorporate them into your daily living.

In addition to these avoidance strategies and preventative measures, there is another very important way to prevent back problems and that is to improve the strength of your back muscles. There is a whole chapter dedicated to stretching and warming exercises that I do every morning and these include some specifically good for the lumbar region. So if you have back problems, seriously consider the following:

- Standing with your feet apart and knees slightly bent, stretch up and backwards then bend over so that your arms dangle down in front of you. Rest in this position for a while then place your hands under your toes (many of you will need your knees very bent to attain this). Slowly start to straighten the knees and concentrate firstly on stretching your upper back then transfer the stretch to your lower back.
- Stand up straight again (slowly) and with your feet shoulder width apart, twist your upper body at the waist (and definitely not at the knees) so that you face towards the left and hold before then twisting in the opposite direction. Repeat a few times.
- Put your hands on your hips and start rotating your hips in a large circle clockwise 3 or 4 times. Then rotate them in the opposite direction.
- Stand up straight and balance on one leg. Bend the knee of the free leg up towards your chest and hold it with both arms wrapped around it. Put the leg down and repeat with the other leg. If you really cannot balance while performing this, carry it out lying down on the floor or on your bed.
- Move your feet quite wide apart and stretch your right hand down to your left foot and back up again. Then stretch your left hand down to your right foot and back up again. Repeat several times.

I also mention later in this book, the importance of weight bearing exercises and this includes some that strengthen the back muscles. There is one very simple exercise that you can do first thing in the morning even before you get out of bed! Lie on the top of the bedclothes on your back and bring your knees up to your chest and put you arms around them. Pull your knees to your chest but the intent is actually to stretch the buttocks away from the lower back so that you should feel the stretch in your lower back. Now, leaving your legs up (holding your knees with your hands if necessary) rock them over to the right, so that the right leg touches the bed and hold. Then do the same over to the left. Repeat right then left as often as you like. If you usually get out of bed with a sore back, you should find a lot of relief from this simple exercise.

There are various gym apparatus and exercises designed for strengthening the back. One that I do not recommend is the so-called dead-lift. This is where you stand feet apart with a barbell on the floor in front of you and bend right over with legs almost straight (some even recommend totally straight – God help you!) to grab the bar. Then you slowly stand up straight with the weight and then bend back down till the bar touches the floor again. This is repeated a number of times. Of all the weight exercises I have ever done, this is the only one that has caused me injury, so I no longer do it! The best equipment I have found is the Lower Back Machine or Chair. You set the weight as appropriate then sit in the 'chair' and bend backwards against the tension to an angle of 30-40 degrees then slowly sit upright again. I usually repeat this 6 -8 times. Not all gyms have these but most have an apparatus called a Roman Chair where you lie face down on a post, body straight, at an angle with respect to the floor. You are supported behind the ankles and under the abdomen. Once positioned comfortably, you bend forward at the waist towards the floor and then use your lower back muscles to pull your body weight back up straight and repeat several times. You can hold weights in your hands if you wish to increase the effort and the movement is similar to the dead-lift but seems to be a lot more beneficial without the side-effects! Other equipment that works your lower back is the cable machine that you can use for a rowing exercise. With sufficient weights on the stack, stretch the cable out by holding it with an appropriate handle while you are sitting on the floor with your heels dug well in. Then lean back until you are lying flat on the floor. Allow the weight to help you sit back up. Repeat several times.

You should realise moreover that strong abdominal muscles also help avoid back problems, so make sure you work on them too – see the chapter on the Abdomen for the Classic Grecian Abdominal Exercises and others that I use during gym workouts. Now I can hear many of you saying things like 'surely I should be resting my back not working it'. Indeed, many years ago this was the common recommendation for back problems but most experts now agree that this is very misguided. Consider for example the conclusions of a 1993 paper which reviewed the literature on bed rest. It found that of the five controlled trials of bed rest for low back pain, the only trial to suggest that bed rest was better than staying ambulant had serious methodological defects. The two most carefully designed and executed trials showed that two days of bed rest for low back pain were better than seven days of bed rest, whereas no bed rest at all was better than four days of bed rest.

One common way to diminish back pain is to have it massaged, particularly if the issue is sore muscles. Sometimes it might be due to a strained, torn or overworked muscle. Or it might be because the muscle has been wrenched at its attachment to a bone. With lower back pain, the attachment point is usually on the pelvic bones and a firm massage here can result in immense relief. This is actually an area that is quite easy to massage yourself and I frequently do so (usually in the shower) if I have been working my back muscles fairly hard. Just get some soap on the edge of your thumbs and forefingers and put them on the very top of each side of your buttocks; then rub firmly up and down. Next make fists and put them higher up, just above your waist and dig in as hard as you can take it and rotate your knuckles in small circles. Keep rotating as you slowly move outwards from the middle of your back to your sides. This is a remedy that you can perform even fully clothed (without the shower and soap of course!)

There are a variety of approaches to body mechanics such as the Alexander Technique, Feldenkrais, Hellerwork, Pilates and the Bowen Technique which appear to assist in back problems (amongst other things). Although I have attended workshops out of interest for some of them and they appeared to be sound, I didn't attend classes long enough to be able to recommend any personally.

Of course, a contemporary cause of problems with the back as well as the neck and shoulders is due to sitting for undue periods at a computer. The main reasons are due to not taking sufficient breaks and appropriate exercise. Some of the recommendations for preventing this are to use a comfortable and adjustable chair such that it is pulled close to the desk with your feet flat on the floor (or a footrest as necessary); work on relaxing your shoulders while sitting as upright as possible; keep your monitor directly in front and at a distance that is perfect for you to see it with no reflections; take a break every half hour to stretch and walk around. Also use some of the exercises described in the chapter on eyes.

One final point on the subject of backs that might surprise or even shock some of you is that I have never been to a chiropractor and in fact I view them with as much suspicion as I do dentists. There is no way that I would want somebody manipulating my bones and joints unless there was unequivocally, without question, no other option – I do not believe that most back problems are anything to do with the bones or joints; they are usually muscular and a massage would be far more beneficial. Most of these problems are preventable by paying more attention to how you move and therefore would not need intervention. Like teeth problems, it is disturbing that the patients that go to chiropractors seem to need to keep going forever. It's worrying that most of the medical profession also seem to view them with some concern.

Interestingly, most of you with bad posture actually know what to do about it – the old adage of shoulders back, head up and chest out really does work. I've been practicing it all my life and the good posture that this develops certainly gives an overall more youthful appearance. Purportedly, Loretta Young the U.S. actress put it this way "Unless some misfortune has made it impossible, everyone can have good posture." and I would add that age per-se is not one of those misfortunes. Frequently, the reason many people find it hard to do is lack of self esteem and that would take a whole new book to resolve! However, the interesting thing is that there are two main schools of thought about making personal improvements. One says, change your thoughts and your actions will change correspondingly. The other suggests that modifying your actions will improve your feelings about things, so by improving your posture, you are likely to improve your self esteem and self image, as well as clearly looking significantly better, younger and more elegant!

Now to gait, which is the manner in which you move on foot. It has an enormous impact on your posture. The two basic human gaits are walking and running. Sadly, as many people age, they seem to think they should no longer run, that somehow it is beyond them. For some folk, it actually is beyond them - regrettably for many, this is because they have not kept up their health, flexibility and mobility when they could easily have done so. Let's face it, you really do look old if you shuffle around, stooped over and unable to move with ease. Even the act of sitting with difficulty and more so, standing from sitting can give the impression of old age even for those that are relatively young. Slumping or falling into a chair is either just laziness or weak muscles and we'll talk about general muscle health in a later chapter. Laziness, I don't intend to bother with here, except to leave you to ponder over whether it is liable to make you look infirm and older.

Many individuals shuffle their feet when walking, they never seem to have learnt to pick up their feet as they walk. As they get older this makes them look much more decrepit than they might otherwise be. Often this shuffling is simply a lazy way of moving or frequently a bad habit started by poorly fitting shoes, especially those with no backs. The answer is simple – just stop dragging your feet and practice lifting them as you walk! Also, start buying properly fitting shoes and no backless ones – flip-flops

(Australian thongs) are particular culprits here. I must say I have a particular dislike of backless shoes, especially thongs or flip-flops since they cause terrible foot muscle problems just trying to keep the things on, let alone encouraging you to drag or shuffle your feet. If shuffling is an issue for you then you should really practice walking in a lively fashion with a spring in your step – it can make you look (and feel) years younger!

Another cause of bad gait which in itself makes the person look old is stooping. Frequently this is a bad tendency which is often developed by taller persons or it might be a pattern developed by poor posture throughout life. Some people suggest that it's a result of their bad back but frankly, stooping or bending over frequently makes a bad back worse as we have discussed previously.

Many victims have a bad gait because of a mechanical problem, such as a leg slightly longer than the other, or due to feet problems. I've seen some miraculous recoveries with the use of orthotics in these cases. However, there are also those who simply damage their own feet by not looking after them. The excess weight that an obese person carries around will surely injure their feet eventually. Not cutting the toenails frequently enough so that they are too long when wearing shoes is a clear potential cause of harm. Of course badly fitting, too tight or too short shoes will also cause problems. If you insist on following fashion so intently that you damage your feet then eventually you are likely to end up hobbling around or with an ageing gait! If you have got trouble with your feet then make sure you include the exercises described further on, especially the chapter dedicated to the feet.

Review of Chapter 6

This chapter looked at how we might improve various types of posture that would otherwise give us an aged appearance. The main causes of back pain were reviewed with suggestions for prevention. Better approaches were recommended for carrying out a number of common tasks. Various useful exercises (for your back and abdomen) were considered which when used could significantly reduce your chances of hurting your back and will improve any aches that you already have. Some massages were described and caution was raised with regards to chiropractors.

Chapter 7 - Your Abdomen and Waist

We are now going to look at how your body shape can make you look older. It is probably obvious that this is mainly associated with excess weight so let's consider a variety of beneficial exercise types to assist here. The other half of the story is what we consume and this chapter will review healthy eating habits with a variety of tips that you might like to follow. With regards to youthfulness, there is no doubt that being overweight definitely makes you look older. Some fairly recent studies in obesity suggest that rather than weight per se, a better indicator of potential health problems is the size of the waist. In fact, waist measurements of over 102 cm (40 inches) in men and over 88 cm (35 inches) in women were determined to be the thresholds for increased likelihood of developing weight related health disorders. Interestingly, at least one study has shown that people perceive a relationship between age and the ratio of the size of the waist to the chest. That is, if you have a large waist in comparison to your chest then you appear to be older. One famous U.S. business writer had an interesting observation – "Middle age is when your broad mind and narrow waist begin to change places."!

So apart from increasing your chest size, which of course, many females do artificially anyway for other reasons and men can do somewhat by weight training, the obvious answer is to reduce your waist size. We will discuss clothes in another chapter but this is certainly one way where you can affect how large your waist looks. In fact with the current vogue of wearing loose, sloppy casual clothes, this is more likely to end up giving the impression that your waist is larger than it actually is! Wearing belts is also clearly another way to hold the waist in somewhat but please, do not be tempted to tighten it so much that most of the excess simply hangs over the top!

Other studies have shown that excess weight and particularly a large waist make you less appealing to the opposite sex. More specifically, research has shown that females rate males more attractive if they have a low waist to chest ratio and men find females more attractive if they have a low waist to hip ratio (apparently less than 0.7 is best!). Prolific research was carried out in this area during the nineties. A rather different take on the subject was carried out at the University of Newcastle in the U.K. They concluded that even more significant is a BMI of about 21 (Body Mass Index – a measure of weight relative to height). The research was studying men's views of female attractiveness and anybody fatter (or thinner) than this BMI was considered less desirable! So if you are already very thin, you might feel justified in moving on to the next chapter!! Some of you will no doubt be bemoaning the fact that not so many decades ago fashions were rather different and a curvy figure was considered very desirable (and still is in some cultures). A certain full-figured British comedy actress was certainly reminiscing about a long gone age when she concluded "If I had been around when Rubens was painting, I would have been revered as a fabulous model. Kate Moss? Well, she would have been the paintbrush."!

So what can be done naturally to reduce the waist size and keep it that way? Well there are three main habits that I have developed -

The first is to exercise regularly. Until recently, the experts recommended that we exercise at least 3 times a week for 20 minutes. Suddenly, this has become 30 minutes a day for at least 5 days a week! Don't get too hung up on these amounts – the important thing is to incorporate something regular and as frequent as possible into your weekly routine. Now, there's no doubt that regular exercise and keeping fit reduces your risk of developing or dying from cardiovascular disease. In fact, research suggests that if you are sedentary and do little or no exercise, you are nearly twice as likely to have a heart attack as someone who exercises moderately. So, if you currently do no exercise, you had better start today! Begin with a small amount and build up gradually. We will discuss a variety of different forms of exercise later but right now we need to understand what types of exercise are useful to reduce weight. Well they include activities such as walking, running, cycling, swimming and rowing. These can be done mostly for free by just getting out there and doing them or you can do many of these things in a health club, albeit in a more artificial way. There are a variety of machines and classes that you can use. I typically perform 20 minutes of aerobic type exercise at the start of my gym workout. I prefer a Nordic ski machine (elliptical trainer) though I sometimes use a treadmill (running machine) or stationary bike. My most popular form of aerobic activity is dancing! One sport I gave up long ago was squash (raquet ball is a version played in the U.S.A.). Like many others that participate in this sport, I was overweight, not really fit enough and only played once or twice a week. It suddenly dawned on me one day that it was an excellent way to bring on a heart attack or at least injure the knees or ankle joints. There are certainly better ways for non-athletes to get fit! So I moved on to less damaging exercise.

There are some misconceptions around about the difference between aerobic and fat burning exercises. It is generally agreed that the more intense you work out, the better it is for the cardio-vascular system and your overall health. However, some authorities claim that for fat burning, you need to tone it down (forgive the pun). So they recommend that you workout at a lower heart rate or intensity to burn more fat.

Although it seems to be true that more fat is burnt for the same amount of effort expended during the exercise period (but note that this means working out for longer since the intensity is less) over a more extended timeframe, there is no difference between low intensity and high. So you might as well work as hard as you can for whatever time you can spend exercising. Despite the prevailing view that aerobic style exercise is best for fat burning, there have been some surprising results that indicate that weight-bearing (or resistance) training can work even better, including for females who often avoid it, mistakenly assuming that it will grow unwanted muscles. For example, an Australian researcher showed that while performing resistance training, overweight pre-menopausal women burnt 50% more fat. He also found that resistance training seemed better at reducing abdominal fat than aerobic exercise. In addition to formal exercise, something else to consider is incidental exercise. In today's world we hardly walk anywhere and most of us work in sedentary roles sitting in an office. Wouldn't it be much healthier and use more calories if we took the stairs instead of the lift (elevator); went outside and played with the children instead of staying indoors playing video games; walked (at least the shorter distances) instead of driving; got up and walked around every so often instead of remaining seated all day (and all night); threw out the remotes and got up to change the TV channels? In fact I believe that the current wave of obesity sweeping the wealthy nations has as much to do with the arrival of TV as it does with bad eating habits. I have no doubt that if you threw out your TV you would lose plenty of weight very easily!

The second way to help reduce waist size is to perform specific exercises for the abdominal muscles. This will not, as some pundits suggest, remove fat specifically from around the waist but it will help to hold-in the stomach area naturally. In addition, with the abdominals tighter, it is also likely to help you eat less. I do exercises for the abs every time I go to the gym (2 – 3 times a week) at the end of my workout. I base my exercises on what an instructor once called the "Classic Grecian Abs Workout". The abdominal muscles actually consist of several different muscles (eg. upper, lower, middle, obliques) and this set of exercises is intended to work out all of them at least once. It consists of the following –

- Lie flat on your back on the floor. I usually start by doing a shoulder stand. This can be achieved by rolling back slightly as you raise your knees above your chest and then push your feet into the air. You can assist this by pushing against your hands but once your lower body is upside down in the air, rest your upper arms on the floor and grip your hands at your hips so as to support yourself. You will now be effectively upside down with your feet in the air, supported on your upper arms and shoulders. It will probably give your neck a good stretch so be careful here! I usually stay like this for a minute or so but the longer the better, if you have time. Some of the benefits of this position are counter-gravitational. That is, many of your organs are now hanging differently; the blood has to flow differently; and your joints (including your vertebrae and discs) obtain relief from their normal weight-bearing stress and so on. If you can do a headstand then the benefits would be even better. You can buy equipment that lifts you up by your feet and leaves you dangling upside down. I have no idea whether they are really useful but I have never seen them in a gym so perhaps this is an indication that they have dubious benefits.

- Now lie flat on the floor again then put you hands flat, palms down, under your hips (this is to prevent a strain on your lower back and in particular to prevent you using the psoas muscles instead of the abdominals). Bend your knees up to your chest breathing out then push your feet almost straight out horizontally breathing in and hold. Repeat this action several times. As you get more advanced, you will find that you can get even more benefit by lifting your head slightly off the floor. If your lower back hurts at all then stop; you might need to adjust the positioning of your hands and also focus your attention more on your abdominals.

- Lying flat again, put your hands, palms down beside your hips and push your feet straight up vertically into the air so that your backside comes up off the floor while breathing out . Hold momentarily then come down to rest on the flat of your back (leaving your legs still pointing upwards) breathing in. Repeat up and down several times.

- Now with your back and head on the floor, bend your knees so that your feet are flat on the floor a short distance from your back-side. Cross your arms over your chest and perform several crunches. A crunch is where you lift your upper back only off the floor, aiming your chest at your knees.

- Proper sit-ups are frowned upon nowadays but I still do them in addition to crunches! After doing only crunches for a long time, I discovered that I could hardly sit up when I wanted to (this first happened in a martial arts class where I needed to get up and out of the way fairly quickly!). The muscles necessary barely worked, so I decided to ignore the apparent experts as I've done several times because if you need certain muscles to do certain actions (like some dance moves or lifts or an activity at work) then you have to strengthen the necessary areas. The other thing is that the 'gurus' keep changing their minds anyway so that something you might have been doing (or alternatively, avoiding) for years is suddenly decided to be different! I do my situps with my hands on my temples. One of the reasons that situps have been frowned upon is that they can tend to use the psoas muscles more than the abdominals and sometimes these might pull on the backbone. If you are concerned, don't do them but I concentrate on my abdominals while doing situps and it has never been a problem; also ensuring that your legs are not straight helps here.

- The obliques are worked by doing crunches at an angle - diagonally towards one knee. First do a set of alternating crunches – left, right, left, right etc. Then do a set of all to the left and then a set all to the right. Don't bother with what some proponents suggest and touch your elbow to your knee, instead aim the left side of your chest at your right knee and vice versa. In particular for many of these exercises, do not strain your head towards your knee as this can affect your neck.

- Now lying flat again, bring your thighs up vertically and bend your knees so that your lower legs are horizontal up in the air. Put your hands at the sides of your neck and crunch upwards so that you are aiming your chest straight up in the air (not forwards). Keep your elbows back and do not pull your hands against your head from behind, otherwise you might put undue stress on your neck joint. Repeat up and down (preferably not touching the floor with your head on the way down), fairly fast, 10 – 30 times.

- That's the end of the specific abdominal drill but while I'm on the floor, there are a few other things worth doing! Firstly, stretch your lower back and abdominals by lying on your back and bringing your feet up a bit towards your backside then arching your back so that your stomach is up in the air – perhaps help to hold it there a while with your hands and arms from underneath. Then stretch your very lower back (and pelvis) by bringing your feet (soles on the floor) right up close to your backside with your knees bent up in the air and roll both legs over to the right (keeping them together) while twisting your upper body over to the left with your arms stretched outwards to that side. Now reverse that position so your legs are over to the left and upper body to the right. Do again 3-4 times.

- Now it's time to roll over onto your front. Then with your hands behind your head, lift the upper part of your body up off the floor and hold for a while. Repeat a few times. This time, leaving the upper body flat, lift your stiffened lower body, from the waist down, up off the floor and hold. Do this several times. Now with your arms out in front, lift the upper and lower body both up, balancing on your tummy (this is called a Superman!). After holding for a while, I then keep my body stiff and rollover to the left front side of my tummy, pause and then move over to the right front side of my tummy.

- Then I stretch my spine by staying on my front and bringing my hands close to my shoulders, palms on the floor and push my upper body upwards, bending at the waist and holding for some time. While doing this, I also take the opportunity to do some neck stretches by twisting my head to the right then to the left a few times.

- Next comes the 'plank', a fairly new but popular exercise that works well for strengthening the abs and the back muscles. Still lying prone, make a fist, clasp it in the other hand and put them on their sides just above your head, resting them on the floor. The sides of your forearms should also be resting on the floor – these two sides of a triangle will be your upper supports. Now push your whole body up off the floor so that you are supported only by your toes and your forearms. Make sure that your body is perfectly straight and almost horizontal – many exercisers incorrectly have their backside sticking up in the air! Hold this position for a count of 10 – 30.

- After collapsing back onto the floor after the plank (!), I suggest that you stand up as follows – put your hands to either side of your head and arch them up onto your fingertips. Push yourself up onto your knees by walking your hands gradually down towards them. Continue walking your hands down till they are beside your knees then push yourself up on to your feet with your fingertips, then stand up. The reason I do this is that it is good strengthening for your fingers and there aren't many exercises for this.

I normally do 8 – 12 repetitions of each of the exercises above. If you are using a gym then there is usually an area for stretching where you should find foam mats to lie on. I usually lie directly on the floor without a mat though certainly on my full-size towel.

The third method to reduce your girth, of course, is to diet, or better still to permanently modify your eating habits. Typically, a diet lasts at most a month or so and then most participants give up and regress to over-indulging and eating unhealthily and they're back to square one or worse. Whoever it was that said "I keep trying to lose weight... but it keeps finding me!" certainly knew the feeling! In my late thirties I discovered that my cholesterol was rather high and I started to review my health. I realised that I was also overweight so I decided to trim off about 20 pounds (about 10 kilos). I did this over a period of a few months and it also resulted in reducing my waist-line by over 5 inches (13 cms). Because of the cholesterol issue, I cut right down on fatty foods. You don't need me to tell you this, it's in most healthy diet books and articles but basically, it meant stopping eating French fries and other fried foods, chips, crisps, cream, butter and margarine, ice-cream and cheese. I also diminished my consumption of meat, especially fatty varieties and certainly trimmed it before eating. Additionally, I reduced considerably starchy foods like pasta, potatoes, bread and rice. Furthermore, I practically stopped drinking alcohol altogether. As the saying goes "Your stomach shouldn't be a waist basket."

But perhaps more importantly, I started to eat large amounts of fresh fruit. This has several advantages for weight loss - fruit has effectively no fat, has relatively low calories and is a natural laxative! I must say that it didn't seem to be much of a hardship especially as the results were fairly quick. I never felt hungry because I allowed myself to eat as much fruit as I felt like. I started to feel much better and healthier than I had ever felt in my life and I have continued with these eating habits practically ever since (just one lapse when I lived overseas for a while but getting back to a fruit diet for a few months afterwards helped sort it out!). During that 'health-kick' period I studied and learnt a lot about better eating habits. Here are some things that I remember and still tend to take note of 20 years on –

- Take a moment to relax and take a few deep breaths before launching into a meal.
- Turn the television off during mealtimes.
- Eat more slowly than normal – savour every mouthful and chew many more times than you usually do. To help with this initially, put your knife and fork down after each bite.
- Use smaller plates so you have less excuse for overloading it with excessive amounts of food. In fact researchers have noted that most people will finish whatever is on their plate no matter what the serving size. With a larger plate and serving spoon, you are likely to dish up over 50% more food than if you used smaller implements!
- Eat smaller, more frequent meals – 5 or 6 a day are typically recommended.
- Have a drink (I don't mean alcohol!) about an hour before and an hour after a meal to help you feel full. Incidentally, I rarely drink during the meal itself.
- If you tend to snack too often, keep only more-healthy items in the cupboards and fridge such as dried fruit, pre-washed and chopped raw vegetables, small fresh fruit (berries, apricots…). By the way, it's surprising how much you will enjoy these 'new' foods and dislike the 'old' ones after you have got used to them, which can take just a couple of weeks or so.
- Do not shop for food when you are hungry!
- Apart from fruit, lettuce is the ultimate slimming food. It tends to fill you up but contains almost no calories. One cup of shredded lettuce has around 20 kilojoules or 5 calories.
- Soup is another good filler that contains few calories.

Eating out can often be a problem for those struggling to keep their weight down and frankly we could all do well to prepare our food at home where we know what we are putting into it. If you must eat out, memorise the following magic phrases which I forced myself to use but now say automatically and with ease –

- 'Please can I have salad with that instead of chips / French fries?'
- 'No cream with that, thanks.'
- 'Can you give me a small portion, please.'

For many individuals, it is not just the wrong foods but they simply over-eat. In some cases, as with the so-called gourmand, they may be eating excellent (in terms of cuisine) food but just quantities that are too large. I have to say that the U.S.A. is the worst culprit here. Having visited a large number of times, I am still amazed (frankly appalled!) at the ridiculously huge portions of food dished up at restaurants (and presumably in their homes also). I assume that this started as a marketing method to encourage customers to patronise certain restaurants which has snow-balled out of all common sense. Of course this is not a new phenomenon. The British aristocrats were famous for their banquets, the Romans for their orgies (including their method of using a feather to tickle the throat to throw-up in preparation for the next course) and the Greek philosopher, Socrates was well aware of his compatriots' excesses when he wrote "Thou shouldst eat to live not live to eat"! I have to confess that I find the temptation of buffets rather difficult to ignore so I generally avoid them. I had a rather disquieting episode with one quite early in life and luckily I took note of it! I was on an overseas trip as a young man on expenses and a group of us went to eat in a Scandinavian Smorgasbord which was upstairs. I ate so much food that I had real trouble getting back down the staircase! It was sheer gluttony but it left an indelible memory as a warning not to over-eat too much.

If you really need to lose weight and are seriously having problems, here's my tuppence worth on the subject of a diet – whatever else you eat, make sure that you have at least five portions of fruit every single day. A portion means a whole banana, apple, pear etc or an open handful of berries, apricots, plums etc. Dried fruit can also be included although like bananas, only one portion a day can count towards these 5 portions (even though you are quite at liberty to eat more of them).

There were two other habits I started, initially as part of the cholesterol reduction regime. One was to eat breakfast regularly and the other was to eat oat bran everyday (on my breakfast cereal). Before that time, I rarely ate breakfast. However, it seems that it helps to kick-start the metabolism into action early in the day plus it prevents you snacking badly during the morning. The cynics suggest that the so-called benefits of breakfast are just PR made up by breakfast cereal companies but I must say it certainly has been helpful to me in my overall well-being and better eating habits. I always drink orange juice as part of breakfast too since vitamin C is apparently an important factor in assisting the body to absorb the iron in the cereal. Oat bran has been shown in several studies to help reduce cholesterol levels. This message seems to have been corrupted somewhat and there are many who eat other types of bran, such as wheat bran which do not have the same effect. In fact, it is also rather sad how the original proposed value of oat bran muffins has been totally negated by the ensuing rise in popularity of all types of other, rather unhealthy fatty and sugar filled muffins!

The fact that fruit is also a natural laxative reminds me of something I heard many years ago regarding keeping slim. The wife of a work colleague of mine was doing some research for her degree into why some of the population were thinner than others. She compared a whole range of possible reasons but the only thing that showed a correlation was that thinner people went to the toilet more often! So, to keep trim, make sure that you go daily, at the very least, or if you are really keen, you can also train your body to go more often. There are those who believe that since you eat at least three times a day then you should also go to the toilet the same number of times. While it is true that we have a gastro-colic reflex which prompts us to feel like going to the toilet whenever we eat, most of us do not respond to it and it is perfectly normal to go once a day. I don't personally feel the reflex much except when I drink coffee – that seems to be a good immediate purgative for me! I'm sure that it would be quite easy to attune your body to pay more attention to the reflex and respond to it, if you so desired. There are also some natural laxatives such as prunes, apricots, figs or rhubarb that could certainly be very helpful in this area! My father used to grow rhubarb and my mother used to make it into jams, pies and crumbles and I still enjoy it today. I have occasionally eaten a portion of prunes in the evening and it is impossible not to go to the toilet early the next day! Other things that are certainly useful to assist regularity are exercise and fibre.

Now I realise that backsides don't exactly come under the heading of Waist and Abdomen but it's not worth creating a special chapter to remind you that a sagging bottom (or conversely, a disappearing, almost non-existent bottom) is extremely indicative of an aging body. The most likely cause of both these afflictions is lack of physical activity of the affected area. That is, insufficient exercise directed at the gluteus maximus. In the chapter on weight bearing exercises, I mention how a Leg Press machine also works these buttocks muscles. Here's some more detail about how to use it - Sitting in the machine, put your feet high up on the plate, wider than shoulder width apart and with your toes pointing slightly outwards. Keep your back pushed into the seat. Move the lever at the side of the seat to release the plate and take the weight. (If you are a beginner then use very light weights.) Lower the plate down towards you until you feel the strain in the back of your thigh (the hamstrings). Push the weight back up to the starting position. Carry out around eight repetitions. Do not allow it to bounce at either end of the movement.

Here's some other exercises that are very good for your butt. They can be done with or without weights – you can hold dumb-bells in your hands or hold a barbell across your shoulders.

Squats

Place feet shoulder distance apart with your head facing forwards. Keep your back straight and do not lean forward. Now bend your knees until your thighs are horizontal, making sure that the weight is pushed down through your heels. Hold for a few seconds then straighten your legs, squeezing your backside as you return to the starting position. Replicate several times.

Walking Lunges

Keeping your back upright, take a large step forward with your right foot. Your knee will be bent and your front shin should remain in a straight line with your ankle. Your back knee should be bent, almost touching the floor with your left foot pointing forwards up on your toes. Now take a step forward with the left leg in the same way. Continue this movement, alternating legs for about eight steps.

Step Ups

Stand in front of a gym bench (or any step will do). Step up onto the bench with your right foot, lifting your left foot up as well so that you end up standing on the bench with both feet. Now lower your right foot down to the floor again, followed by your left foot. Do this again but this time start with your left foot first, followed by your right. Repeat several times.

Other approaches that I have heard are good to help redefine your buttock area are pilates and yoga.

While slightly off the subject, let's go back to the chest. There is no doubt that many females bemoan the loss of tautness in their breasts as they start to sag. Similarly males look in the mirror at their undefined, weak looking pectorals and dream of a barrel-chested look. Well the situation really need not be so dire as this – there are some simple exercises that both sexes can carry out to improve the situation. Many women must remember the schoolgirl slogan "I must, I must, I must improve my bust" as they carried out a form of isometric exercise for their pectorals by squeezing their hands together at chest level. Well it's never too late to start this up again! The chapter on Weight Lifting Exercise describes some machines specifically designed for the chest as well as some stretches. Others appear in the chapter on Daily Stretches. Of course the classic exercise for the chest is the push-up and you should be doing these several times a week if you wish to rejuvenate the appearance of your chest or bust. Females typically perform push-ups with their knees on the ground instead of coming up on their toes. But anyone who finds it difficult to do full push-ups could use the kneeling method. Here are two other exercises using free weights which are designed for the chest -

Bench Press

Holding dumb-bells or a barbell, sit on the end of a bench then lie back ending up with the weights just up above your chest. Now position your hands to the sides of your chest with your elbows down under the weight. Push (press) the weight straight up keeping your elbows to the sides until your arms are extended but do not lock your elbows. Lower the weight back down to the upper chest. Repeat several times.

Lying Dumbbell Flyes

Holding dumbbells, sit on the end of a bench then lie back ending up with the weights just up above your chest and your feet firmly on the floor. Making sure that your bottom, back, shoulders, and head are positioned firmly on the bench, push the dumbbells straight up above you. Prepare the starting position with your elbows slightly bent and your palms facing each other so that the dumbbells are touching each other. Keeping your elbows slightly bent, slowly lower the dumbbells away from each other in an arc until your hands are out either side of your body and you can feel a comfortable stretch in your chest area. Raise them up in the same arc back to the starting position. Perform this several times.

Review of Chapter 7

This chapter has been concerned about the size of your abdomen (or more specifically your waist) because several studies we looked at have shown that it can affect how old you appear. The role of exercise generally was considered to ensure staying healthy plus a number of different types of exercise were suggested to reduce your waist measurement. These ranged from aerobic to strengthening your abdominal muscles. In particular we went through the Classic Grecian Abs Workout. The other important area addressed was diet, including some revision on those foods that we all know are fattening and refreshing our memories about those that are beneficial. The positive effects of fruit were especially reiterated. A number of approaches to eating and useful habits were suggested. We also strayed outside the specific subject and considered ways to rejuvenate our buttocks and chest areas.

Chapter 8 - Your Legs, Knees and Feet

We've talked in a previous chapter about how poor gait, shuffling and generally hobbling around can make you look older and in this chapter we'll discuss some ways to look after your feet which are frequently the cause of these problems. This will include some specific exercises; the effects of excess weight (a common theme); harm that can be caused by certain shoe types; and some simple ways that I care for my feet. Arthritis, the dreaded affliction of the knees and other joints will be addressed with some investigation as to how to avoid it and relieve it. We will also review the issues of cellulite and varicose veins in the legs.

It's quite amazing how far some of us are prepared to go to follow shoe fashion despite knowing that it is damaging our feet; we will wear badly fitting shoes, ones that are too tight or backless ones that we have to strain to keep on our feet. Then of course, females wear high-heeled shoes even if they're killing them! No doubt there's no point in my going into a tirade about how you shouldn't do this because it might catch up on you later in life! At least I will remind you that prevention is better than cure. It might be worth you going back to the chapter on gait where I have discussed some of the issues regarding poor shoes.

Once again, excess weight is an enemy here. For many, the extra strain put on the legs and feet causes immense damage, including fallen arches and varicose veins. So keeping the weight down is clearly sensible.

There are some simple exercises that will strengthen the ankles, feet and toes. One often mentioned is to practice picking up a crumpled towel or other objects with your toes. Another that I frequently do is as follows –

- With your feet slightly apart, come up onto your toes as high as possible and hold for a while then stand back down again and then lift the front of your feet up so that you are standing on your heels. Hold for a while and keep repeating at least ten times.

However, even before doing strengthening exercises, it is wise to stretch and warm your ankles and other joints in the feet. This will help keep them flexible which will improve your walking (and running etc). Remember that there are 26 bones in each foot so that's also a lot of joints! The following are incorporated into my daily morning stretch and warm-up exercises (the full set of which are described in a later chapter):

- Stand on your left leg and bring your right knee up towards your chest. Move your foot from left to right about ten times then move it up and down about ten times. Next rotate it clockwise about ten times then the same anticlockwise. Now shake your foot somewhat before putting it back on the floor slightly behind you up on the ball of the foot and stretch the toes by bending them. Then tuck the toes under and stretch them the opposite way.
- Now redo everything with the other foot.

Be sure to let me know how much relief you find from these exercises.

If the skin on your feet is unhealthy, diseased or damaged in some way then naturally this is likely to affect your ability to walk in an elegant or youthful manner. The feet should be washed regularly, especially between the toes and they should be dried completely – it is amazing how many bathers do not dry their feet properly and walk around with damp feet – a sure-fire way to encourage fungal growth and other skin issues around the toes. Just jumping in a shower or bath of itself is not washing the feet; they need to be washed as you would your hands. Some experts go even further. One, for example, concludes that athlete's foot does not occur amongst those who usually go barefoot - it is moisture, sweating and lack of proper ventilation that cause athlete's foot to grow. According to another, bare feet get the beneficial fungicidal effects of the sun's ultra-violet rays. If you do catch tinea or the like then it is quite easily eradicated with any one of a variety of fungicidal creams but do take note that you need to keep applying it for several weeks, even if it seems to have cleared up. Apparently this is due to the fact that even though the adult fungus may have been killed there can still be spores waiting to germinate.

It is worth mentioning here that I have never used deodorants or antiperspirants anywhere on my body. Strictly speaking a deodorant is just another smell (a fragrance or perfume) used to mask any potential body odour, while an antiperspirant contains numerous chemicals designed to block up your pores so that they cannot perform their function of perspiring. These include aluminium chloride, aluminium chlorohydrate, and aluminium-zirconium compounds which react with electrolytes in sweat to create a gel which plugs up the duct of the sweat gland. As it happens, over time, most deodorants have now come to contain many of these same substances. Marketing of these products has been intense and most of the population seem to have been convinced that they really do smell badly and need to use them. I have never believed this barrage of nonsense – in reality there are very few people who smell from perspiring unless they don't bathe sufficiently or rarely clean their clothes. Anybody who does smell probably has some physical condition that needs medical attention. Now that doesn't mean that I don't occasionally splash some cologne on myself if I'm rushing out to a function but I have no intention of clogging my skin with dangerous chemicals. I also find it very objectionable being near somebody spraying this stuff into the air – the bad effect on your nostrils gives a clear feel of how unhealthy the habit is and I have to say that ironically the odour is never a pleasant one!

So here we have a product designed to seal up the pores so that the body cannot eliminate toxins naturally nor cool itself down if necessary. This can lead to the kidneys starting to overwork, potentially leading to disorders in this organ. Natural oils are also prevented from carrying out their function of feeding the skin; so instead of a healthy glow you could end up with pimples. The most dangerous chemical to our health in antiperspirants is Aluminium, a poison which has been linked to Alzheimer's disease. Other research suggests a likely link with breast cancer. At a UK University, they observed that aluminium salts, which exert oestrogen-like effects, promote the growth of breast cancer cells in the laboratory. You should also be aware that some studies indicate that it enters your lymphatic system far easier when you've just shaved under your arms. Unfortunately, even perfume alone has its own dangers. It too can contain dozens of artificial chemicals and some data indicates that in the U.S.A. alone, millions of known asthmatics have attacks triggered by fragrances.

Massaging your feet fairly often will also pay big dividends –in the shower as well as at other times. If you watch the TV at all then this is a perfect time to work on your feet! Alas, there are many who cannot get to their own feet, either because of overweight or lack of flexibility. If you are one of these then perhaps it should be a wake-up call to improve your general health! Even so, it shouldn't prevent you getting attention from somebody else. Personally, I massage my feet most mornings in the shower. This includes firmly massaging all my toes and the bottom of each foot then also the tops of my feet and ankles. In particular, I massage in between my toes and the ligaments all the way up the feet. I have to say that I have no corns or bunions or other issues with my feet, presumably a good indication of how paying basic continual attention to your feet can ensure they are healthy. Toenails that are too long are obviously another detrimental factor in the way you walk! I tend to cut mine every month or so and certainly aim to keep them just below the level of the end of the toe.

Returning to the subject of walking around in bare feet, there is a school of thought that this is one of the best ways to keep your feet in peak condition. They encourage it in all activities including hiking in the countryside. I've never gone that far but I must confess that since moving to Australia where it is common, I usually go without footwear in the house and in my own garden (and of course at the beach, being a popular Aussie pastime!). In fact, according to one paediatric orthopaedist, "Children with the healthiest and most supple feet are those who habitually go barefoot."

Perhaps I should state that many of us have one leg or one foot slightly longer than the other. Apart from the effect of this in itself, it can often additionally cause damage to the hips. If you suspect these problems then getting advice about orthotic footwear might help tremendously. Often, this only means a small insert like an inner sole.

Varicose veins have a tendency to make your legs look old and in fact half the population aged over 50 are affected. They are commonly found on the backs of the calves or on the inside of the leg. It is the job of your leg muscles to pump your blood back to your heart. Valves in the veins prevent the blood from flowing backwards. However, blood can leak back down the vein if a valve weakens or is damaged. If the blood pools then the vein enlarges and becomes varicose. If the varicose veins are severe then other health problems can ensue such as sores, ulcers, swelling and rashes. Acute blood pooling is called venous insufficiency and this could lead to infections and blood clots which are potentially life threatening.

In addition to just age, the chance of developing varicose veins could increase due to hormonal changes such as those occurring during pregnancy, and menopause or due to taking medication such as the pill containing oestrogen or progesterone. Other factors are obesity; insufficient exercise; as well as prolonged standing. However, the exact cause is not clear. It seems that there is no relation between varicose veins and crossing the legs, diet, sunbathing, waxing the legs or tight clothes.

In order to avoid the aging effect of varicose veins on your legs you need to consider observing the following–

- Keep your weight down so as to avoid undue stress on your legs.
- Exercise your legs regularly either in the gym or by walking or running.
- When sitting, elevate your legs. Get up every half hour and move around.
- Don't stand still for long periods. Occasionally sit down if possible or at least move around.

- Avoid tight clothing from constricting your legs or waist.

The above will also ease the discomfort of existing varicose veins as will wearing elastic support stockings.

There are a variety of medical treatments that are used to deal with them which apparently have high success rates. A natural supplement that seems to be efficient is horse chestnut extract. Even the prestigious Mayo Clinic acknowledges that research indicates that horse chestnut seed extract may be beneficial in decreasing size, pain, itchiness and fatigue and that it may be as effective as compression stockings.

One other condition affecting the legs that just about everybody, especially females dread is cellulite! It's intriguing but it seems to me that twenty years ago, it only appeared to apply to clearly overweight persons. Now it looks as if even many otherwise slim females are afflicted by it. It seems that contrary to popular belief, cellulite is not related to obesity, since it occurs in overweight, normal, and thin women. Yes, this is an almost exclusively female affliction because their adipose tissue under the skin is structured differently from men. However, there are still some males that develop the condition, usually due to a hormonal cause. The word cellulite is not strictly a medical term. It was coined in France over a hundred years ago to describe those deposits of dimpled fat and has been used commonly in Europe for many years, whereas it only came into parlance in the U.S.A. in the nineteen seventies. It should not be confused with cellulitis, which is an infection of the skin and its underlying connective tissue.

There are many misconceptions about the composition of cellulite such that ironically large numbers of claimed treatments are asserting they are curing things that don't even exist! Frequently it is alleged to be an improper combination of fat, water and toxins that the body has been unsuccessful in eliminating. However, medical authorities agree that it is just ordinary fatty tissue. In one double-blind study, specimens were collected of regular fat and 'cellulite' fat with a needle biopsy and analysed. No difference was found between the two types. The dimpling effect occurs because there are fibrous tissues connecting the skin to deeper layers and which also create partitions that contain fat cells; when fat cells increase in size, these sections bulge and produce the infamous waffled appearance of the skin.

There are huge numbers and types of so-called cellulite-curing products available that prey on females' desperation. These include supplements containing herbs and minerals; loofah sponges; mitts and washcloths; creams, gels and liquids; toning lotions; massagers; impregnated pants; brushes; rollers and body wraps. In addition, all sorts of treatments, costing hundreds of dollars can be undergone from machines that heat or vibrate or stimulate muscles electrically; to injections of enzymes or hormones; as well as special massage treatments. Most claim to reduce the size of the thighs and buttocks despite the fact that even if it were true, this in itself, of course has no bearing on whether what remains is still dimpled or not!

Here are some facts about some of these processes that you can review and decide for yourself - Iontophoresis devices are used to introduce ions of certain medications into body tissues for therapeutic purposes. Muscle stimulators are used for some genuine medical reasons also. However many health salons are alleging that they can also use them to perform face lifts, reduce breast and abdomen size, as well as remove wrinkles and cellulite. The FDA (Food and Drug Administration) in the U.S.A. has concluded that claims about muscle stimulators or iontophoresis equipment being able to carry out any type of body shaping or contouring is fraudulent. At one infamous trial as far back as the seventies, they were able to prevent sales of the devices, which furthermore, the judge concluded could cause miscarriages and aggravate many pre-existing medical conditions, including hernias, ulcers, varicose veins, and epilepsy! The U.S. Federal Trade Commission has taken other legal action successfully against many marketers of claimed cellulite reduction products including tablets, creams, tables, body wraps, briefs and so-called 'institutes'.

Many salons are promoting body wraps that are claimed to trim down multiple parts of the body. Typically, the assertion is that the water-logged fatty tissue is melted away! As noted above, this description of cellulite is nonsense. Perhaps the treatment might cause temporary water loss as a result of perspiration but this would be replaced in no time by drinking. Moreover one needs to seriously question the notion that herbal wraps can detoxify the body. Firstly, cellulite contains no such toxins; secondly can such topical applications really penetrate into the tissues anyway? As for pills and tablets, we need to be aware that no product taken orally can cause reduction of a specific part of the body. As already noted, cellulite is not the result of toxins or fluid build-up so any product claiming to eliminate these does not understand the problem; and doesn't this appear to be most of them? Many well-meaning souls proclaim the healthy powers of large intakes of water. I'm glad to say that there are medical experts that agree with me that it is an erroneous concept that drinking more water will help any skin condition (unless of course you are truly medically dehydrated). Moreover since toxins do not cause cellulite then drinking more water cannot eliminate them!

Interestingly, in 1998, the FDA approved a certain massage tool with motorized rollers with a suction device that compresses the body tissue in a process that the company called Endodermology. However, within a year, the FDA ordered the promoter to stop claiming that it could have more than a temporary effect on cellulite. Even then it usually takes dozens of treatments to get any results, and one or two maintenance treatments per month are required otherwise such effects are soon lost. Some independent studies have found no changes at all, others have claimed a reduction around the thigh of just under half an inch (one centimetre). This doesn't sound very significant to me, especially as it is only temporary; is it? Bear in mind also that reduction in size doesn't necessarily equate to removal of cellulite!

The intervention of liposuction is claimed by some proponents to be of assistance. However, this technique of extracting fat by vacuuming it from under the skin is apparently not effective for cellulite. In fact, liposuction could make the appearance of the skin worse by sucking out the cushion of fat lying just beneath the skin so that even more dimpling occurs. Sadly, hormone therapy doesn't seem to treat cellulite either, even though female hormones appear to play a role in contributing to the condition.

We need to realise that despite all the hype about expensive (and non-functioning) products, the amount of fat in the body is largely determined by our eating and exercise habits. Perhaps heredity plays some part in determining how the fat is actually deposited around the body but the reduction or prevention of fat of any type can be accomplished only as part of an overall weight control program.

So if the most effective way to tackle cellulite is to take the same approach to lowering weight and overall body fat generally then we are back to the tried and true approaches mentioned in several other parts of this book; namely -

Eat a balanced, healthy, low-fat diet with piles of fresh fruit and vegetables.

Keep your heart pumping with regular exercise at a gym or power walking, swimming, cycling or dancing.

Include exercises that specifically target the thighs and buttocks.

So I'm sorry that I could provide little news about genuine cures of cellulite apart from healthy living! However, here's a trick which is apparently used by makeup artists on film stars! It appears that cellulite tends to be less noticeable with darker skin. So, if you have a light skin tone, try to conceal your cellulite using a self-tanning product (or if you prefer it work on the real thing – with care).

We can't go past the subject of legs without mentioning your knees. If they are damaged or not very strong then there is a high likelihood that they will factor in to making you look old and crotchety. We have been conditioned to expect that as we age then we are likely to get various forms of arthritis. The sad news is that there are many in the population who are starting to show signs of this problem in their thirties and even twenties! So the issue is not merely age. According to the medical experts, the best ways to avoid bad knees leading to possible surgical replacements are weight maintenance and low-impact exercise – what a surprise and a recurring story with almost every subject we cover! Apparently, just being five kilograms over your ideal weight can double the risk of arthritis in the knees and it seems that the majority of knees that need medical treatment are due to this ailment. Osteo-arthritis is the term for it from degenerative or wear-and-tear causes. What tends to happen is the surface layer of cartilage breaks down and wears away so then bones under the cartilage start to rub together. This can cause pain and swelling and also loss of motion of the joint. In long term situations, it could also create disfiguring of the affected area. The joints usually affected are neck, lower back, knees, and hips, as well as fingers and thumbs.

So what if you already suffer from this condition; what can be done to cure it? Well there don't seem to be any foods that are naturally helpful although there are those who swear by fish oils (these might take many weeks before benefits are manifested). There are some foods that might be aggravating for many folk, so it is worth avoiding them and seeing if it helps. These include citrus fruits, milk, tomatoes and potatoes. Unfortunately, one of the impacts of the sometimes chronic inflammation is that cytokines are produced. This together with side-effects of constant medication can lead to a variety of nutritional deficiencies, so it is vital to eat well and perhaps take mineral and vitamin supplements. More surprisingly, the pharmaceutical industry has little to assist, apart from with the associated pain. Glucosamine is getting a lot of publicity right now though no scientific studies have yet been conclusive. A large number of studies seem to show that glucosamine (as well as chondroitin) is effective in helping with arthritis and other joint problems. This includes regrowing cartilage, pain reduction and reduced swelling. Glucosamine is produced naturally by the body. Every supplement company seems to have released a product in the last few years! Omega 3 essential fatty acids are also associated with relieving arthritis symptoms – they have significant anti-inflammatory properties. They are found in fish, flaxseed (linseed) oil, rapeseed (canola) oil, walnuts, and dark green leafy vegetables. Supplements also exist; most being cod liver oil. Regular use and exercising of the affected joint certainly appear beneficial, including swimming. You should also massage the area frequently (or better still get somebody else to massage you – always a pleasure). A positive attitude is certainly helpful as well as a sense of humour such as that shown by the Chicago man who at 93 was told by his doctor that he had developed osteoarthritis in his knee and that it was a result of aging. The quick reply was "My other knee is 93 years old too, and it doesn't hurt at all."

And what about avoiding it in the first place? Interestingly, various studies, including a significant one carried out by Johns Hopkins University in the US, showed that much depended on what you did in your twenties. In particular, indications were that staying at or below ideal body weight when you're young decreases the risk of osteoarthritis in the hip and knee. Conversely, excess weight seemed to increase the risk. This is assumed to be because the overweight creates greater stress on weight-bearing joints. It should be noted that increased muscle mass at the hips and knees can stabilise these, which could be a good way of reducing the likelihood of arthritic damage. Other activities that can be carried out during our youth that seem to help lower the chance of getting arthritis are, not surprisingly, regular exercise; eating a balanced and nutrient rich diet; and avoiding stress and damage to the joints.

There is no chapter particularly dedicated to your hands so I will just note here that they are a frequent indication of a person's age even if the rest of their body looks young. Usually this is due to the same issue affecting other areas of the body; simply that the muscles near the skin are atrophying. Similar to the Facial Isometrics, this can be alleviated by exercising the hands as described in the chapter on daily stretches. Of course, it also helps to pay attention to your nails (and the ends of your fingers generally) by keeping them clean and trimmed as well as attending to any damage. I'm sure I don't need to also mention that continually holding a smoking cigarette will surely damage and age your hands.

Review of Chapter 8

If your feet are rather weak then you might work on the exercises described to improve the flexibility of your ankles and toes, as well as general feet strengthening.

It might be appropriate for you to consider the damaging effects that excess weight might be having on your feet.

Some of you will undoubtedly benefit from reviewing the types of shoes you wear.

Some of the simple ways that I described to care for your feet could be useful.

A fair amount of information was provided about varicose veins and cellulite, together with the best approaches to help avoid these ailments.

If you suffer from arthritis, whether in your knees or elsewhere, you could be interested in returning to this chapter to explore the issues of food, supplementation, weight and exercise that I weighed up.

I also threw in a small paragraph about keeping your hands looking youthful!

Chapter 9 - The Clothes You Wear

"Clothes maketh Man" so the saying goes. Of course this refers to females as well as males. The clothes you wear can have a tremendous effect on how outdated and aged you look. Now I am not going to recommend that you look like "mutton dressed as lamb" but if you are still wearing clothes that you bought ten years ago just because they still fit or haven't worn out, then chances are that they are looking extremely old-fashioned! Also insisting on wearing something that is "comfortable" or a "favourite" when it is rather worn or faded is likely to be a giveaway of your age and a lack of fashion sense! What frequently happens is that many get stuck in the dress style of the time period when they felt most stylish, typically when in their twenties. So clearly they are going to look outdated if they keep hanging on to these fashions.

Colours are something that tend to be associated with certain decades or eras. Also, the height of the waistline of clothes cycles up and down throughout the decades! In the mid-00s, you may not feel right (or look right) in bumster fashions but you certainly shouldn't have waistlines way up to your ribs nor the bottoms of your trouser legs up above your ankles! Of course hemlines are continuously moving up and down. Watch out when wearing shorts; you should have noticed that nobody wears socks pulled up to the knees anymore. Similarly with swimwear, are you still wearing small swimming trunks when everybody else is wearing boardshorts?

Those of all ages can have bad or unfashionable dress sense but it seems to be more noticeable the older you are. So men, stop wearing socks with sandals; consider wearing your shirts outside rather than tucked-in; buy the more casual option; sport longer shorts; don't wear belts on your shorts; checkout the latest in eye-wear…. Go clothes shopping with a younger person and take note of their advice! However, do not go overboard and try to dress like a teenage child! Some adults do this and they just look silly not younger. Another approach is to take note of what celebrities your age are wearing. Perhaps read fashion magazines every now and then to get an idea of what's new and youthful. But again the idea isn't to look like an adolescent. Instead you should aim for a look that's contemporary and stylish. Let me know about any other examples you are aware of.

If you are into the very common mode for females of wearing extremely body-hugging tights with a sloppy T-shirt on top, you might like to look in a full-length mirror and reconsider whether it really is a youth enhancing ensemble. This form of dress has the extraordinary ability to fail on two paradoxical counts – wearing clothes that are too tight can be very unflattering (for males and females) especially if you have some excess fat; wearing clothes that are too baggy can make you look bigger than you really are! A very important rule as you grow older is to select clothing that suits the shape you are right now, not how your body shape was several years ago. Even the ancient Greeks were aware of this concept. It was Euripides the Greek poet who is credited with noting "Know first who you are; and then adorn yourself accordingly."

If you are responding to all this with thoughts like "but I feel more comfortable with my existing clothes" or "but that's the way I've always dressed" well it's up to you if you really want to look younger! It can also make you feel better if you dress well, a fact that has been known for centuries; for example Charles Dickens once wrote "Any man may be in good spirits and good temper when he's well dressed." The finest recommendation here is to buy less articles but of better quality.

I have to finish off this chapter by saying how important I believe it is to dress for the occasion. I was horrified when I first arrived in Australia to find patrons attending the theatre in shorts, T-shirts and thongs (the flip-flop shoes not the underwear!). It is a fundamental rule of success to understand what to wear in what company. Thomas Fuller, the seventeenth century British clergyman and author had some recognition of this when he opined "Good clothes open all doors." But it is more than this – you need to be casual or comfortable if the situation dictates but you also need to fit-in or impress in other circumstances.

Review of Chapter 9

Some of the specific issues of dress mentioned here include –

- Looking out of date.

- Wearing worn-out clothing.

- Various examples of old-fashioned styling, such as the height of your waistline.

- Discussion of colours.

- Being aware of preferring baggy and comfortable favourites.

- Dressing for the occasion.

There are many people who age simply because they expect to. They decide that there are certain things that they should not or cannot possibly do and guess what – after a short time they can't. They create little conversations in their head saying things like "I must act my age" or "I'm too old to do such and such". Well I have no such belief system and I am still doing things that many individuals much younger than me have already decided that they are too old or incapable of doing! The impact can be even more severe when these types of phrases are spoken out loud and repeated. Another issue of mental attitude is when old crocks resort to the view that "in my day things were so much better". Well I'm not sure what 'your day' was but the reality is that you are right in the here and now not somewhere else. All that sort of reminiscing certainly makes others think you are old. It also starts to make you act and look old. As one American author put it "We seem to be going through a period of nostalgia, and everyone seems to think yesterday was better than today. I don't think it was, and I would advise you not to wait ten years before admitting today was great. If you're hung up on nostalgia, pretend today is yesterday and just go out and have one hell of a time."

We've all met hypochondriacs and there are those who become so as they get older. They convince themselves that they have to expect to get aches and pains and even certain diseases. Well again, surprise, surprise, since they believe it then it starts to manifest for them. Frankly my motto is - as long as you don't abuse it (too much) and you use it then you won't lose it! Certainly you should expect to be fit and healthy all the time and probably you will be. Meditation and affirmations can certainly help your frame of mind here. It's more than just thinking positively – it's about knowing that you are healthy and capable and then acting that way. I set myself some affirmations in this area and repeat them frequently, especially while meditating several times a week. I review them and if necessary modify them every few months. Checkout the chapter on meditation, affirmations and visualisation for help here and with using affirmations in other areas of your life. If you suffer from a severe health problem then I hope that you will find that some of the techniques described in this book can help you. If they do, please send me the details; I'd love to hear about it. There are many other resources on the subject in books and the internet. We can all take some comfort in the advice of the famous U.S. actress who overcame a debilitating stroke while believing that "A strong mental attitude will create more miracles than any wonder drug"

We talk quite a bit about good health in this book but the ability to age well and feel good about yourself also has a lot to do with an optimistic outlook, a good attitude and other effective coping skills. As somebody once quipped "Don't let ageing get you down; it's too hard to get back up!" Some important factors that can help ensure that you have a positive mental attitude as you mature are: being involved in social and community activities, as well as participating in hobbies and socialising. There are a whole range of leisure pursuits and other activities that you can get involved in to keep your mental attitude youthful such as –

- Studying and practicing a foreign language.
- Learning to dance, play a musical instrument and/or sing better.
- Tending a garden.
- Studying.
- Starting a business.
- Doing charity or other voluntary work.

Music can often be a huge divider of the generations. You've heard the catch-cry "if it's too loud, you're too old!" But give modern music a chance – play it and listen to it. Only ever playing (or liking) the music of your own teenage and 20s years is a sure age giveaway!

It might sound too simplistic to some of you but it really pays to be 'young at heart' that is, to feel young and to act young. This includes being accepting of music, clothes and other activities of today's youth. Do things that younger people do and go to places where they are. As the Nike ad puts it so well "Just do it". Mix as much as possible with them but preferably in situations where they are treated as equals. An alternative is to spend as much time as possible with your grand-children especially as they get older. Of course, one way to feel younger is to date a younger mate. There's a famous phrase that comes to mind – "A man's only as old as the woman he feels" and of course this can be turned around to apply to women also. Naturally, these types of relationships need careful consideration as there might be corresponding drawbacks and pitfalls. I am certainly not recommending this approach to already married individuals!

There is a huge amount of information about positive thinking and if you have never studied any then I recommend that you do learn about its benefits. Somebody with a positive mind anticipates happiness, good health and a successful outcome of situations and events and whatever the mind expects, you can be sure it will find. So what can you do to develop a positive attitude? Try the following -

- Smile more often.

- Use humour; watch comedy shows; laugh at yourself and the world. Put up on your wall the following quote allegedly from Katharine Hepburn "Life can be wildly tragic at times, and I've had my share. But whatever happens to you, you have to keep a slightly comic attitude. In the final analysis, you must not forget to laugh."
- Have confidence in yourself and mix with other positive people.
- Read inspiring stories and quotes.
- Simply choose to be happy and look at the bright side of life. If nothing else, for the sake of a youthful appearance, remember that constant frowning contributes to expression lines and eventually wrinkles!

Abraham Lincoln once said "Most folks are about as happy as they make up their minds to be." Negative thinking is simply an attitude that is a habit. These current habitual attitudes are created over time by the feedback of parents, friends, society and ultimately by yourself. They form our self-image and our view of the world. These attitudes are largely maintained by the inner conversations we constantly have with ourselves. An important step in changing our attitudes is to change our inner conversations. Positive Thinking is a simple tool that helps us to change this negative thinking. A recently concluded 10-year study showed that pessimistic men were twice as likely to experience angina and heart attack as optimistic men. Recall Winston Churchill's apparent words – "A pessimist sees the difficulty in every opportunity; an optimist sees the opportunity in every difficulty."

Review of Chapter 10

Some of the specific issues mentioned relating to a positive mental attitude included:

- Avoiding saying out loud or to yourself such phrases as 'in my day'; 'I'm too old to do X' and 'I must act my age'.
- Beware not to develop hypochondria as you get on in years – expect to live a long, healthy life.
- Use meditation and affirmations.
- Work on generating an optimistic outlook and a good attitude as well as other effective coping skills.
- Consider getting involved in social and community activities, as well as participating in hobbies and socialising.
- Keep young at heart and mix with younger groups.
- Give modern music, fashion and culture a chance!
- Study and practice positive thinking.

<u>Chapter 11 - Regular Exercises</u>

One of the main tenets of this book about looking younger naturally is to exercise regularly and to carry out a variety of different and specialised exercises. In this chapter, I simply mention the different types of exercise that I carry out and the frequency. The specifics are covered in other chapters. The health and longevity benefits of exercise are not newly discovered; the ancient Greeks didn't create the Olympic Games for no reason. Hippocrates, the physician still respected to this day and who gives his name to the Hippocratic oath that doctors take, wrote "All parts of the body which have a function if used in moderation and exercised in labours in which each is accustomed, become thereby healthy, well developed and age more slowly, but if unused they become liable to disease, defective in growth and age quickly." Also Plato, the renowned thinker, asserted that lack of activity destroys the good condition of every human being, while movement and methodical physical exercise save it and preserve it.

If you are not yet convinced that you should be exercising more, here are some of the youthful benefits of regular exercise that you should be aware of:

- Improves & strengthens your immune system.
- Gives you extra energy.
- Reduces stress and improves the ability to relax.
- Helps relieve headaches and other pain.
- Reduces back problems and improves posture.
- Lowers your cholesterol and triglyceride levels.
- Helps lower depression.
- Improves balance, flexibility and co-ordination.
- Increases bone density and helps ward off osteoporosis.
- Boosts mental alertness.
- Improves digestion.
- Reduces the chance of heart disease.
- Reduces blood pressure.
- Improves skin tone.

By the way, one important point while exercising is not to hold your breath but to breathe naturally. As a general rule, you should breathe out when tensing to lift or move something as well as when compressing your midriff and inhale before lifting or while expanding your midriff.

Morning Stretch and Warm-up

As the name suggests, I perform these every single day in the morning. I remember reading about a Russian gymnastics coach who after much research had concluded that the best way for athletes to warm-up was to do it first thing in the morning and that this was even more important than warming-up just before a specific physical activity. I have been doing these exercises every morning for as long as I can remember and I have to say that I have never sprained or strained any muscles or joints. My balance is extremely good and the stretches mean that I am quite flexible. I strongly recommend that you also incorporate these exercises into your daily routine – they only take about ten minutes to complete.

Daily Facial Isometrics

We have already covered these in a previous chapter. Although this says 'daily', I probably do this whole group of exercises about 4 – 5 times a week. It takes about 6 – 10 minutes in total and usually I carry them out while I'm doing something else so there's no excuse for you not to have enough time for them! Anyway, if you want to look younger, what's 6 minutes a few days a week?

Weights and Aerobic Exercises

There is a special chapter devoted to this. I usually go to the gym 2 to 3 times a week where I do about 20 minutes aerobic exercise and 30 – 40 minutes of weight training, followed by abdominals. In addition, I dance a lot – perhaps 2 or 3 times a week, which is more aerobic exercise. Of course, you don't have to go to a gym to be able to carry out aerobic or weight training exercises. Any article or book that you read about being healthy will state that you need to do a certain amount of physical exercise for good health and weight control. So you really should consider getting going with this and just make the time necessary. There are plenty of other far less useful activities you can replace, such as sitting in front of the TV. This reminds me of a man who said to his wife "I want you to know that I would not want to live in a vegetative state being supported by some machine. If that ever occurs, please disconnect it." So his wife went over to the wall and unplugged the television.

Aggression Relievers

Relieving stress is vital for good health and is particularly important for keeping you youthful. One form of stress relief is reducing the aggression that can grow over time. This can cause a build-up of harmful hormones in the bloodstream. Simple activities such as driving can create aggression and stress which is never allowed to dissipate properly. Instead of turning this anger and aggression against other drivers, or your fellow humans, or family it is more healthy to take it out on a punch bag or better still to take up a fighting sport such as boxing or martial arts.

Back

Unlike most of the population, I never get back aches so I strongly recommend that you start doing all the different types of back exercises and stretches that you will find in this book. Most are included in the Daily Stretches section and in the Gym Workout as well as the specific chapter on the Back, of course. However you will find a few others scattered throughout other sections including the simple one I mention that you can do while still in bed!

Eyes

The chapter on eyes describes exercises that I was typically doing every day, though I do them less regularly now that I definitely have to wear glasses to read. However, there are other exercises that I frequently do while still in bed if I want to wake up quicker or if I've been reading or working at the computer too much. These would also be useful if you get eyestrain at any time.

Scalp Massage

In the chapter about hair, I describe the importance of scalp massage to help prevent hair thinning. Effectively, I do this every day when I wash my hair. One or two days a week I might not use shampoo but I would still massage my scalp.

Posture Correction

I frequently remind myself about my posture. Am I standing tall? Is my head up, my shoulders back and my chest out? Am I lifting my feet as I walk?

Review of Chapter 11

In addition to describing the many youthful benefits of exercise in general, this chapter mentioned the following types of exercise that I carry out and the frequency:

- Morning stretches, joint warm-ups & balance.
- Daily facial isometrics.
- 2 to 3 times weekly weights & aerobics.
- Aggression relievers such as martial arts & punch bag.
- Various back exercises.
- Frequent eye exercises.
- Daily scalp massage.
- Continual posture correction.

Chapter 12 - Daily Stretch and Warm-up Exercises

I stretch my muscles and warm-up my joints every morning without fail. I have been doing this for many, many years. I am certain that this is one of the main reasons that I am pretty fit, very well and perfectly healthy. I never have back pain or headaches. I never have stiff muscles or problems with my joints. If you want to feel youthful and look sprightly then you really need to consider performing the simple exercises in this chapter regularly. You would then soon find that you will not suffer from the aches and pains that seem to afflict so many as they get older (and some not so old!). The other main benefits for you are that your overall flexibility will improve tremendously so that you will feel and move as if you were years younger, your joints will be far more loose and less painful – if you suffer from arthritis or stiff joints, you could be amazed at the improvement. Stretching your spine, especially your lower back will give you renewed vigour. I know there are those who find it tough to even contemplate physical activity but I advise you to heed the words of Edward Stanley, Earl of Derby who was a British politician some centuries ago. He said "Those who think they have not time for bodily exercise will sooner or later have to find time for illness." First thing in the morning is the best time to stretch and warm-up. Not only does it prepare your body for the rigours of the day but it also kick-starts your metabolism at the start of the day. Many practitioners recommend yoga as a good stretching activity. I cannot comment since I have never studied it.

All of these activities are carried out standing up – there is no need to get down on the floor. If you are too incapacitated for even that then you can adapt some of them to be done while sitting in a sturdy chair or perhaps while lying on a bed. If you are not used to exercising then please take care – start slowly and with small movements at first building up to fuller motion over time. Perhaps you might prefer to start by working with somebody else to help you with your balance and the more strenuous stretches (this person is typically called a 'spotter' and is commonly used by body builders and weight trainers so don't feel embarrassed). It may be that you are unable to perform some of these exercises fully. However, don't use that as an excuse to give up – either leave that particular one out or better still modify it slightly or work on it so that over time you are able to achieve it. So let's start at the top, with our head and work downwards:

- Firstly, neck exercises which were described in the chapter on the neck. These should be done fairly slowly and gently. With your hands on your hips, and holding the shoulders, arms and upper torso still (and your shoulders down & relaxed), start by twisting your head gently to the left (and remember what you can see there), now twist it the opposite way to the right (and remember what you can see there). Now repeat to the left but try to see a bit further around. Do the same to the right. Repeat this a total of about ten times. You might hear a slight crunching sound as you twist your neck around – this means you really need this exercise! Do not use your hands to help push your head further than you can naturally twist it as this might cause some damage. This method of stretching to a point then coming back and stretching a bit further, I call "Progressive Stretching".

Next, lay your head down to the left so that your left ear comes close to your left shoulder. You probably will not be able to touch your ear on your shoulder but this is fine. Now lay it over to the right side. All the time, keep facing forwards. Repeat this a total of about ten times.

Now, hang your head down forwards gently so that your chin comes down towards your throat. Again, you might not be able to touch it but that's OK. Lift it back up straight. Repeat this a total of about ten times. Finally, hang your head down forwards so that your chin comes down towards your throat again and now roll it from left to right. Do this about ten times.

- Hang your arms down the side of your body and lift your shoulders up then rotate them around several times. Rotate them back the other way several times.

- Work on the finger joints by slowly rolling the fingers and thumb into a fist then open them out and stretch them out flat as hard as you can. Repeat in and out several times. Next hold the hands out horizontally with palms facing towards each other and stretch the fingers one at a time downwards, working the finger joints that are closest to the hand and then upwards. Perform several times. Now rotate the hands clockwise at the wrists several times then back in the opposite direction. Put the palms of your hands together in front of your chest and push inwards especially the ends of the fingers so that you are stretching your fingers back. Work on each of your finger joints so as to relieve and preferably avoid any arthritis by massaging each joint with the forefinger and thumb of the other hand. Next use your palm to bend the opposite wrist as far as possible downwards then upwards. Finish by letting the fingers and wrists go loose and shaking the hands back and forth, as well as up and down.

- Moving to the elbows, hold the arms out from the body and rotate the forearms at the elbows clockwise then anti-clockwise.

- Now working on the shoulders, rotate the arms at the shoulders in large circles in one direction several times then in the other direction. Hold the arms out horizontally in front of you then bring them back without twisting the arms so that when they arrive outstretched at the sides, you can feel the tension against the joints and muscles. You need to avoid yanking backwards too hard which might strain the joints and muscles so do not swing them back (this swinging method of stretching is called 'ballistic' and is not recommended, especially if you are inexperienced, since it can tear muscles, joints or tendons.). Carry out several times then do the same thing but diagonally so that the right arm moves up slightly and the left downwards. Reverse the action, so the left is upwards and the right downwards. Now replicate again with the arms equally horizontal but this time swing the arms back and twist at the shoulder so that the arms go behind your back and preferably touch the hands behind your back. After repeating several times catch the hands together behind your back and hold before slowly pulling the arms upwards as far as you can. Then still behind your back, hold the left wrist with your right hand and pull it slowly across to the right. Reverse hands and do it in the opposite direction. These latter stretches are mainly for your chest muscles (pectorals).

- Next we stretch the triceps (the muscles on the opposite side of your upper arm to your biceps). Lift up your right arm and put your hand behind your head and as far down the left side of your back as you can. Now lift your left arm up putting your hand on your right elbow and push your arm gently further down your back. Repeat with the other arm. Stretch your upper back and shoulders (and triceps differently) by bringing your right arm horizontally across your chest then raise your left arm up vertically just above your right elbow and pull your right arm further into your chest and out to the left and hold. Carry this out with the opposite arms.

- Moving down to the midriff, leave your left arm hanging at your side and touch your right hand gently against the right side of your head. Now lean sideways to the left feeling the right side stretching. Note how far your left hand gets down your body. Change hand positions and repeat by leaning to the right. Now repeat to the left attempting to stretch past the previous point (Progressive Stretching). Do the same to the right. To increase and slightly modify the stretch, hold both arms up above your head and grab your right wrist with your left hand then pull it over to the left. You should feel a good stretch in your right side. Perform the same thing over to your right and repeat both several times. Now do the same thing except pull slightly forward and to the side.

- The following sequence will be of benefit to the midriff, back, legs, internal organs and hair! Hold both arms up above the head and stretch back slightly; then bending at the waist and with the knees slightly bent, throw your arms down and backwards so as to flex your lower back, then hang down there for a while so that the upper half of your body is effectively upside down – this will stimulate lots of the organs inside and get the blood flowing more in the upper half of your body. Come back up slowly and replicate this action and then while hanging down, start tapping and pounding gently on your head, and using your fingers encourage your hair to hang downwards. This will improve the blood flow in your scalp and to your hair follicles. After a while, put the fingers of your right hand under your right foot and the same with your left. Slowly straighten your right knee as much as possible so that you are stretching the back of your right leg as well as your back. Now do it with your left leg. Finally straighten both legs as much as possible! Stand back up slowly.

- Now concentrate on warming up your hip joints by waggling your hips from side to side with largish movements. Then proceed to rotate them in one direction and then in the other. Keeping your feet apart and slightly splayed open (to avoid excessive strain on the knee joints), knees slightly bent and your hands on your hips, twist your upper body to the left. Hold; then twist to the right. Perform a few times. Now twist again to the left but this time turning the feet also and bending the left knee. Do the same to the right and repeat a few times so that the knee joints are worked. Now do the same thing again but this time concentrate on stretching the calf of the rear leg – you can assist this stretch by keeping the rear knee straight and pushing back/down on the ball of the rear foot and making sure this foot is turned in slightly. Feel free to assist yourself by pushing off your leg with your hand to stand back up, if necessary. Continuing to work on your hips (and also your back), start a slow marching action where you bring your knees up as close to your chest as possible.

- Next we will move down to the knees again. Firstly lift the right knee up and wrap your arms around it, pulling it towards your chest (this is a good stretch for your back and will also help you to keep your knee high for the exercise which follows).

- The following set is aimed at warming up the knees and ankles but it is also very good for your balance. Having good balance is a very important part of staying youthful. So start by raising you right knee up towards your chest and maintaining it as high as possible (not with your arms or hands). If you start to lose your balance, bend your left knee slightly to lower your centre of gravity (if you are having serious difficulty with this then stand close to a wall which you can touch for support when needed). Sweep your lower right leg slowly from side to side at the knee then rotate it around from the knee clockwise a few times then in the opposite direction. Finish off by kicking your leg up as high as you can in front of you but make sure this is not a 'ballistic' uncontrolled swing that might strain the muscles. Instead raise it up with the power of your muscles. Put your right leg down then do it all again with your left leg. Now we'll work in the same way on the ankles (twist left and right; then rotate clockwise then anti-clockwise) but instead of doing a kick, simply move your foot up and down at the ankle. Finally the toes - shake your foot somewhat then put it back on the floor slightly behind you up on the ball of the foot and stretch the toes by bending them. Then tuck the toes under and stretch them the opposite way. These latter stretches are described in the chapter on Feet.

- The next sequence is a bit more advanced but you should work on perfecting it since it is very good for your flexibility and balance. Standing on your left leg, lift your right foot up behind you and catch it with your right hand. Pull it as far up and as close to your backside as you can then hold for a while – do not let the knee flare out to the side. Then without putting your foot down, move your knee forward before pulling your right foot out to the side so that your bent right leg is as horizontal as possible. Then again without putting your foot down bring it from out on the right side across to the left side and hold your right leg up as horizontal as possible with both hands. Finally (again without putting your foot down), take your right foot with your right hand and straighten your leg out as much as possible diagonally to the right in front of you. Then replicate all that with your left leg. Many of you will find much of this very difficult to do. However keep working on it and over time you might surprise yourself! If you really cannot keep your balance, practice balancing with one hand touching a wall or chair. The first stretch is for the quadriceps (front of the thigh) which is an important muscle so if you cannot grasp your foot or ankle then do it with a towel wrapped around the ankle and the ends held with the hand.

- I finish off with a workout for the back and hip joints (These latter are based on splits and might be too advanced for many people but the initial back stretches will be invaluable to all). Stand with your feet quite wide apart and stretch your right hand down towards your left foot (and touch it if you can) then without coming up, twist across as you stretch your left hand towards your right foot. Carry out back and forth several times. To stretch a different part of your back (and to increase the stretch for those that can), continue by trying to touch the right elbow on the ground then the left and so on. With the knees bent, put the fingers of both hands under your feet then slowly straighten the knees as much as possible as you pull gently against your feet, firstly concentrating the stretch in your upper back then moving it down to your lower back. Now for the splits – if you are doing this on your own and feel the stretch is too much or you cannot get back up then simply fall over onto your backside and get up from there! Otherwise, continue with your legs wide apart and facing forward, put your hands down in front of you (I vary this with palms down or up on my fingers or on my knuckles) then slowly allow your feet to slide outwards and hold for a while (side splits). If you're feeling up to it, try and touch your head to the floor. Then bring your left foot back in towards the middle so that you can bend your left knee and twist your body around to face to the left before stretching the left leg back out in front of you as you put your hands on either side of your body (front left splits). Stretch as far as you can and hold. If you're feeling up to it, try and touch your head to your knee. Push yourself up as far as you can then very slowly twist around to face to the right and repeat the stretch (front right splits). It is very important to come out of this very carefully and gently so bring your front right foot back as close to the middle as possible, bending the knee then bring your left foot in also. If your backside is up in the air, bring it down towards the ground then use your leg muscles to stand up.

You will have noticed that several of these exercises rely on your balancing ability and indeed as you practice them you will dramatically improve your stability. As many get older they frequently get more unsteady on their feet. Apart from physical disorders such as damage to the inner ear, this problem is mostly due to not participating in relevant physical activity – a case of use it or lose it. If you don't want to look old, feeble and doddery then it is essential that you improve your balance. Let me know your progress with these.

Sounds like far too much to squeeze into your morning while rushing to get ready for work or get the kids to school or whatever? Well once you've got into the routine, it only takes 10 minutes to complete the lot! In fact, I reduce the time even further by carrying out two sets of exercises at the same time where feasible – for example some of the hand exercises with the feet exercises. Frankly, this is probably the most important 10 minutes you will spend during the whole of the day (apart from doing your facial isometrics!).

Review of Chapter 12

It is recommended that the exercises described in this chapter be carried out every morning so that you will start to feel alive, dynamic and full of energy. They will keep you flexible and protect your joints and muscles so that you will be able to move more easily including walking and running. They will also improve your balance. You will almost certainly get relief from stiff and sore neck and back problems as well as countering arthritis.

Why should you bother with weight bearing exercise? Well there is no question that a toned body helps you look more youthful. We have already discussed how a trimmer waistline helps you appear younger and 'gym-work' should also be part of your regular regime to be generally fit, lean and healthy. Another important factor is that without weight bearing exercises, your muscles are likely to atrophy and this shrinkage will create flabby skin – a certain indicator of aging! One particular area that tends to get flabby, especially for women is the underarm, which is the triceps muscles. So I certainly recommend that females take notice here, as well as the stretches aimed at triceps. Of course, it goes without saying that weight training will make you stronger generally. But perhaps the most important general health reason for many of you is the huge benefits that resistance training provides for your bones.

The three most important forms of exercise are stretching, aerobics and weight bearing (including isometrics for muscle toning). In this chapter I will describe some of the major weight bearing exercises that I do regularly, usually in a gym but you can just as well do many of them at home with or without specifically designed equipment. However, since there is so much home gym equipment lying around unused, I would highly recommend that you join a gymnasium and schedule specific times with yourself or a trainer if you can afford it – it is so easy to put off exercising at home when there are so many other 'vitally important' things to do around the house instead.

I have already talked a bit about aerobic exercise in the chapter on your Abdomen and Waist. I usually do 20 minutes of aerobic activity on a machine such as a Cross-Trainer (a.k.a. Elliptical Trainer or Nordic Skier) or treadmill or bike as a warm-up before starting my weight bearing activities. It is also considered good practice to stretch the muscles after you have worked them out. Many of the stretches already described in the chapter on Daily Stretch and Warm-ups would work but I will also describe some more focussed and directed ones that I do in the gym.

Many of you will have noticed that a person's muscles seem to shrink as they get older. In fact generally, muscles reach their maximum size at about age twenty five then start reducing in size. This shrinkage becomes even more significant over the age of fifty. Research done in Sweden shows that it is indeed the number of muscle cells, or fibres which decline with age but it turns out that it is only fast-twitch fibres, not slow-twitch that disappear. Moreover, individuals who carry out weight training can even grow their slow-twitch muscle fibres. By the way, slow-twitch fibres are those which contract slowly but have longer endurance, whereas fast-twitch fibres contract powerfully and rapidly but have limited endurance. The research also explains that the reason for the fibre loss is due to the gradual deteriation of motor nerve cells which connect them to the central nervous system. But the good news is that with weight bearing exercise you can prevent and even reverse these muscle fibre losses. In addition, weight training will increase the number of capillaries in your muscles which will help increase your strength.

One special subject to consider here is bone health and strength and its bearing on osteoporosis. The word osteoporosis is based on Latin, meaning "porous bones." There seems little doubt that regular weight-bearing exercise is the best approach to ensuring healthy bones and reducing your risk of developing osteoporosis as you get older. Apparently about two million Australians are afflicted with osteoporosis (about 10% of the population!). I assume that if you had it then you would move around very cautiously, looking decidedly aged, yet a natural way to prevent it is readily available – it just takes a little effort and time to carry out some weight bearing exercise. Bones are comprised of about 35 per cent collagen for flexibility and 65 per cent calcium phosphate for hardness. It might sound incredible but apparently our bones are 'broken down' by osteoclast cells to release calcium for use in body metabolism during the day; then at night, while sleeping, they are built up again and weight bearing exercise lets the body know how strongly it needs to rebuild. This process is called "resorption" - areas of bone are dissolved over several days, leaving small holes. Osteoblast cells rebuild the bone, first with collagen and then hardening the bone with calcium and phosphorus. In adults, around a third of our bones is replaced each year. Osteoporosis is when the bones over time do not rebuild properly. This causes them to become thin and brittle so that they break more easily.

Certain foods can provide vitamins D and K, essential fatty acids, calcium, and magnesium that are essential to maintaining good bone health. For calcium eat dairy products, canned sardines, salmon, and dark-green vegetables such as cabbage, kale, and broccoli. For magnesium eat brown rice, whole grain cereals, fruit, vegetables, legumes, and seeds. It seems however, that you need to correctly balance the amounts of calcium and magnesium to protect against osteoporosis (and heart disease). In fact, those who intake high amounts of calcium but with a low consumption of magnesium are at a higher risk of heart disease than those who do not take calcium at all. The best way to increase levels of magnesium is by eating more vegetables and fruit. One study which observed men and women over 40 found those with the highest fruit and vegetable consumption had the strongest bones. On the other hand it seems to be advisable to avoid soft drinks. These contain large amounts of phosphorus, which can apparently deplete the bones of calcium. So osteoporosis is a likely outcome for heavy imbibers of soft drinks.

Make sure that you checkout and compare all the gyms and health clubs within a reasonable radius and also ask about special offers and prices as well as payment options that suit you. If you only want to use the weights and machines room but none of the other facilities then ask for a reduction. Many clubs have pensioner rates though often at restricted times. Indeed, one important point to checkout is the opening times, especially evening and weekend closing. Also, ensure that parking is freely available. More importantly, you should decide what facilities you might be interested in taking advantage of, so you need to be ready to ask whether they also have a pool, spa, sauna, crèche, changing rooms, free and easy parking, fans, air conditioning, etc. Are classes included in aerobics, yoga, martial arts, stretching? Are the facilities clean? Is some personal training advice included? Is massage available? Would you like somewhere to relax afterwards and perhaps socialise a little with other members (not common!)? Make sure that you get a walk-around to see and checkout those facilities. Also ask for a free trial to be certain that the clientele and equipment is to your liking. Make sure you do not take this visit during the quiet periods. One other small word of advice – make sure you checkout what others are wearing to the gym. You don't want to stick out like a sore thumb, especially if your idea of how to dress comes from your memories of your high-school PE classes! The only other items you need for the gym are a bottle of water to be drunk throughout and a towel to put on the equipment (or to wipe it down after using) as well as to wipe your brow!

For many years I did pretty much the same exercises each time I went to the gym, one session concentrating on my lower body and the next on my upper body. After some advice from a trainer, I now change the actual exercises and the order every 3 months or so – it seems the body gets quite used to a routine and needs a wake-up call every so often! There are many books, magazines and websites dedicated to this subject so, as an introduction, I will simply restrict myself here to mentioning what I have found to be some of the more important exercises and leave you (and the advisor at your chosen gym) to decide what actual ones are best for you. The amount of weight that you use is also up to you. It might not be very heavy if you are just keeping generally fit but as you progress you will want to use heavier weights so that typically you will use enough weight that you can only complete the desired number of sets. Sometimes you might increase the weight with each rep (repetition) other times you might decrease. There are a multitude of experts in the field all with different views, so try a few of the different approaches to get a taste of what actually works for you. Perform all motions fairly slowly and in particular do not rush the return (or reverse) action.

Lower Body

I acknowledge that squats and lunges with free weights are probably the best exercises there are for the legs. However, it is easier to use machines and so, for the lower body I use the Leg Extension machine to work the quadriceps (front of thigh) and the Leg Curl machine (I prefer the standing machine to the one that you lie face down on) for the hamstrings (back of thigh). I then use a Seated Calf machine for the Calves. I often also use a Leg Press machine to further work the quads (and also, it works the hamstrings and Gluteus Maximus or buttocks). While on this machine it can also be used to work the calves. I usually include my lower back in this session and this is extremely important as you get older and anyway if you want to help avoid back pain. There are only a few exercises that can be used here and most are rather advanced. I do not recommend the Stiff Legged Deadlift – if performed incorrectly (which is quite common) you can do more harm than good! The best exercise is a specific machine that you sit in and lean backwards against a force that you can modify. Another method is a piece of equipment (Roman Chair) that you lie in at an angle and bend forward at the waist. You come back up lifting you own body weight. As your back gets stronger you can do it holding a weight.

Upper Body

There are many dozens of exercises for the upper body which include the back, chest, shoulders, arms and hands. Here are some of the major ones that I do at the gym. Each is repeated 8 to 12 times.

Biceps Curl (Standing)

Using free weights (a barbell or dumbbells), start with your arms down the side of your body and lift the weight up until your forearms are vertical with palms facing up. Lower to original position. With barbells you can do both arms together or alternate arms.

Triceps Curl (Standing)

These are the muscles at the back of the arm. I usually lift a dumbbell up high, straight above my head with both hands and then keeping my upper arms close to my head, slowly lower it behind my head, keeping my upper arm vertical all the time and simply bending my elbow. I then return the weight to above my head. Another good alternative is to use a cable machine where you stand with your upper arms permanently down the sides of your body and pull the bar downwards by straightening your arm down towards the ground and then allowing the weight to pull your forearms slowly back up by bending the elbow.

Shoulder Press

There are many muscles in the shoulder and many exercises therefore to work them. This press is done by holding a barbell or dumbbells with hands on each side of the shoulders with elbows below the wrists and then pushing straight up until the elbows are not quite locked and then returning to the start position. One particular shoulder muscle that you might like to strengthen is the trapezius. This is located on the very top of the shoulder and is actually part of a much bigger muscle that is a trapezium shape on the back. I call them 'the luggage carriers' because they are the ones that many of us tend to strain a bit when carrying heavy suitcases so if you are going away for a while, you might like to work on them for a month or so before leaving! You can do this by holding some fairly heavy dumb-bells in each hand and shrugging your shoulders upwards.

Forearm Curl

Many experts suggest that there is no need to bother with specific exercises for the forearms since they are also worked by most other arm and shoulder exercises. I'm not sure of the veracity of this so try holding a barbell or dumbbells with the bar permanently horizontal and hold it out with your palms up so your upper arms remain fixed against your sides and the forearms are horizontal. Now let the fingers of the hands drop downwards then lift the weight up again and bend the wrists up and towards your chest. Different muscles are worked by doing the reverse forearm curl, that is, holding a barbell out with palms facing down and bending the elbows as you lift the weight up and towards your neck then lowering it back to the horizontal starting position.

Chest Press or Flye

While there are many exercises that can be done with free weights and benches here are two machine exercises that might be better for beginners. Sitting on the Chest Press machine, grasp the handles and slowly extend your arms forward till the elbows almost lock then allow the arms to move back again. A Pec Deck Squeeze Machine allows you to effectively do a Fly (Chest muscles are called pectorals or 'pecs'). Sit on the seat with your forearms behind the pads and your upper arms horizontal. Start by squeezing out and inward toward the front and centre of your body. Hold elbows as close together as possible then return slowly to starting position.

Back

I've mentioned the lower back in the previous section. For the upper back, I tend to use a Seated Row Machine. These come in various forms but typically, while sitting up straight, a pad against your abdomen/chest holds you in place while pulling handles towards the sides of your body. I am not referring to a Rowing Machine here which tends to be used more for aerobic exercise although of course it does also work the back. Another very popular machine that concentrates on the latissimus dorsi (the muscles that show at the side of the upper back giving that much loved triangular shape!) is the Lat Pull Down Machine.

Now having completed you weights workout, which should last at least 30 minutes or so, you need to stretch the specific muscles you have just worked. This might look like a lot of effort but in fact all your stretching will be complete in about 5 minutes. Some instructors recommend stretching immediately after each weight exercise, so do whatever you prefer. Here's a flavour of the sorts of stretches I do:

Legs

Find a pad or bar as high as you feel comfortable (probably around waist height) and lift one foot up onto it then gently lean your body towards it so as to stretch your hamstring. Repeat with the other leg. The quad stretch is included in the Daily Stretch and Warm-up but to repeat it here - standing on your left leg, lift your right foot up behind you and catch it with your right hand (some suggest the opposite hand). Pull it as far up and as close to your backside as you can then hold for a while – do not let the knee flare out to the side. If you really cannot keep your balance, use the other hand touching a wall or chair. Also, if you cannot grasp your foot or ankle then do it with a towel wrapped around the ankle and the ends held with the hand. Many experts recommend various alternative methods while down on the floor. You should already have stretched your calves on the calf exercise machine but I usually do more stretches by finding a block of wood or the lower frame of a machine and standing on it with the balls of my feet. I then push one heel at a time down towards the floor with my body weight.

Arms

For the biceps, stand next to a machine that has a vertical bar of some sort at shoulder level and standing at arms length from it grasp the bar with your palm facing backwards, so your thumb faces down. Move your body forward of your hand so that you can feel a stretch in your biceps. You may need to vary the angles a bit to feel the best stretch. I stretch the triceps at the back of my arm with the same method in my morning stretches - Lift up your right arm and put your hand behind your head and as far down the left side of your back as you can. Now lift your left arm up putting your hand on your right elbow and push your arm gently further down your back. Carry out with the other arm. You can stretch your forearms by bending your wrist forward and gently pushing it down with the other hand then pushing it to one side and then to the other. Finally, push the hand backwards as far as you can.

Back, Shoulders, Chest

Stretch your upper back and shoulders (and triceps differently) by bringing your right arm horizontally across your chest then raise your left arm up vertically just above your right elbow and pull your right arm further into your chest and out to the left and hold. Replicate with the opposite arms. Other parts of your back can be stretched by holding both arms out in front of you and pulling one of them forward with the other hand; while the lats are stretched by holding both arms up above your head and grabbing your right wrist with your left hand then pulling it over to the left. You should feel a good stretch in your right side. Perform the same thing over to your right and repeat both several times. You will already be performing this every morning. There are many other back stretches mentioned in this book, particularly in the chapter on the Back! At last we are at the end with a stretch for the chest. I do this by using a machine again that has a vertical bar, this time higher than my head. I put my arm out to the side with my hand about head high and palm facing forward. Twist your body gently away from your hand as you feel the stretch across your chest.

Just about every time I visit the gym I also workout my abdominals and I have already described this sequence in the chapter on the Abdomen (The Classic Grecian Abs Workout). This takes 5 to 10 minutes; so your total gym visit lasts about one hour.

One of the frequent scourges of getting older is arthritis. Of course, exercise is also very beneficial for your joints (unfortunately, the opposite view was prevalent some years ago). Exercise reduces joint pain and stiffness, builds strong muscle around the joints, and increases flexibility, range of motion and endurance. The morning stretch and warm-ups are ideal in helping here as well as these gym exercises. If you have severe joint problems such as arthritis then of course you might build up gradually. If you are really reluctant to exercise because you are in such pain then you might want to start with water exercises. While in the water, buoyancy reduces stress on your body and makes it less heavy.

If there are times that I cannot get to the gym such as when I am travelling, I have a series of isometric exercises that I can use in the car or in an aeroplane seat. Obviously, some of these should not be done while actually driving. So here's what you can do sitting in the driver's seat – you can modify some of them (particularly those using the steering wheel) if you are in a different seat or in an aeroplane. Incidentally, while flying, I also get up and do many of the 'Daily Stretches' as well as walk around every so often to avoid the dreaded Deep Vein Thrombosis. I hold each tension for a count of about 15 – 20. In some of the descriptions, I mention using both hands or both feet at the same time – if the situation dictates then only do one at a time or wait until you are stationary!

Upper Body

With both hands gripping the top of the steering wheel, palms down, push your hands down against the wheel then pull up against it. Gripping tighter, pull both hands outwards; then push in. Next push against the wheel, forcing your back into the seat, and then pull at the wheel (with a different focus, this can also work your upper back). Finish by twisting your hands out and then inwards. Do similar isometrics at the sides of the wheel (quarter to three position) and at the bottom. Put your arms straight up into the air and push against the roof. If you have a sun-roof or other protrusion, pull your hands forward against it and then back. If it is open you might be able to pull down on it. Push one hand against the door frame and the other against the central section. Pull both hands inwards against the sides of the seat. Hook your fingers under the seat and pull upwards. Push both hands down on the edge of the seat. Put your hands up beside your head and grip the back of the head-rest pulling forwards (with a different focus, this can also work your abdominals). Then put your hands at the front and push it backwards. Put your hands behind the back of the seat at waist height and pull forwards. Put your elbows down tight against your body and push them back against the seat. Put your right hand against the side of your head and push against it (perhaps only a count of 5); then do it with your left. Push your right shoulder against the back of the seat then your left. Then push the whole of your upper back against it. Do the same with each hip and lower back. Finally push each of your hips downwards one at a time.

Lower Body

Bring your calves right up close to the edge of the seat, lifting your feet off the floor then pull your lower legs hard against the seat. Put your feet back on the floor and push forward against your heels. Go up on your toes and push again. Alternately lift up your toes then your heels. Push your feet against each other hard. Hook one foot over the other then try to pull them apart sideways. Put your feet against each side of the footwell and push outwards away from each other. Put your feet under a pedal each (or other protrusion under the dash-board) and lift them upwards. Put your knees together and push against them. Just lift both knees up as high as you can and hold for a count of 20 to 30.

You may have realised that some of these exercises are redundant in that they work the same muscles as previous exercises, so please feel free to prune out any that you do not fancy!

Review of Chapter 13

Weight bearing exercises are vital to prevent muscle atrophy, to keep strong, to tone the body, and especially to strengthen the bones thus reducing your risk of developing osteoporosis.

We started by considering some important aspects about finding a gym and what types of exercise are important.

We touched on specific exercises in some detail for legs, back, arms, shoulders, chest and abdominals.

Then we reviewed some important after-workout stretching activities.

Finally, I described some isometric exercises that I carry out if I am travelling (or stuck in the office!), especially on aeroplanes or on a long car journey.

We have already mentioned in several previous sections about the benefits of managing stress and combating its effects. Stress is perfectly normal in moderation and in fact can be quite useful if directed appropriately. Stress responses are one of our bodies' best defences against dangers. In such situations our body releases stress hormones that instantly make us more alert and focused. The body prepares itself to act with increased strength and speed and the senses become sharper and ready for action. Research suggests that stress can definitely increase our performance - instead of wilting under duress, it can be used as an impetus to achieve success. It can stimulate your faculties to delve deep into your true potential and sharpen your performance. On the other hand, if you are unable to cope with some of the many pressures of life then the outcomes can be very detrimental. As we have discussed in previous chapters, it can certainly affect us in many ways both mentally and physically, subsequently causing us to age prematurely. So right now we will review some of the multiple causes of stress and look at a few of the significant effects that can result but bearing in mind that there is quite a difference between how each of us reacts to the same stressors. I will then give you a flavour of some of the various methods and techniques that I personally use to relieve and manage stress. Considering that he lived to a ripe old age (despite his appalling cigar-smoking record!), we should certainly take note of the words of George Burns, the U.S. comedian, when he supposedly said "If you ask what is the single most important key to longevity, I would have to say it is avoiding stress, worry and tension."

The origins of stress are numerous and include health problems, workplace pressures, demanding relationships, traffic snarls, deadlines, family tensions, financial problems, house moving, divorce, death, unemployment, conflict, prejudice and bullying. Smoking is another factor – objective research shows that contrary to smokers' belief that smoking helps them relax; it actually heightens tension, irritability and depression, especially during the frequent nicotine depletion in the body. Sometimes you can simply avoid these stressor situations but usually you cannot. Some individuals cope better than others and even seem to thrive when times get tough. In the case of work, tense relationships and other situations, for most of us it is definitely wise to instil the habit of taking sufficient breaks. The common recommendation for those of us in fairly sedentary jobs is to stand up every hour or so and stretch. But whatever your occupation, it would be sensible to recharge for 5 or 10 minutes after working hard for an hour. Since a change is as good as a rest, perhaps you might switch to a different project. Either way, you should be much fresher for it. It was Thomas Jefferson who noted over two centuries ago "Nothing gives one person so much advantage over another as to remain always cool and unruffled under all circumstances."

The effects of stress are many and varied – it can cause headaches, low energy, chest pains, muscle weakness, eating disorders, allergies, insomnia, lethargy, low libido, depression and mood swings, backaches, frequent colds, fatigue, poor concentration, hypertension, asthma, diabetes, digestive problems, skin complaints, heart ailments and even cancer. Frequently unpleasant emotional feelings are generated such as inadequacy, depression, anger, fear, worry, tension, aggression and dependency. Such stress and anxiety can be very detrimental to our immune system. A constant condition of strain can result in a loss in neural and hormonal balance. This deficiency will cause increased oxidative damage thus accelerating aging in our body. These chronic disturbances in body homeostasis ultimately affect our hormone secreting glands, cell repair and collagen in our skin and connecting tissues. Recent research also suggests that long-term exposure to adrenal stress hormones may prematurely age the brain. So stress can cause serious physiological effects on the body. Under such nervous tension, your body produces a hormone called cortisol. Normally, this is not very harmful. But with continual or chronic stress, cortisol is secreted excessively and in larger amounts it is extremely toxic. Too much cortisol actually kills and disables your brain cells and can be responsible for forgetfulness, mental haziness, and confusion that are also associated with aging.

The compound DHEA (Dehydroepiandrosterone), a steroid hormone is the natural counter to cortisol since it is secreted by the adrenal glands during buoyant times and it reduces the effect stress will have on you. Unfortunately our capacity to produce DHEA declines with age. Research shows that DHEA also boosts the production of sex hormones and provides numerous health and rejuvenating benefits. A study published in 1998 looked at DHEA's effects on aging. Participants were tested for this hormone's levels and also took cognitive and strength tests. Those with the highest amounts performed better on both assessments. The authors also concluded that those with higher DHEA levels appeared younger. So how can you raise your levels? Well, the natural approach is by reducing stress and thus lowering levels of cortisol. DHEA supplementation is apparently available but it is certainly not recommended without first seeing a doctor and having blood levels of the hormone checked. In fact you need to be aware that many experts are voicing considerable caution about prescribing it for cosmetic uses.

The important point to remember is that the factors mentioned above are stressors not really the cause of stress. The anxiety is actually caused by you; by how you react to those stressors. So the foremost way to address stress is to have a variety of management techniques, preferably preventative approaches. You never know when one of these situations might suddenly occur so you need to be pre-prepared. You also need to keep yourself in a relatively calm state so as to be able to face the continual small stressors rather than allow them to gradually build up to a crescendo. This was well put by the U.S. journalist who wrote "The time to relax is when you don't have time for it."

So what are the activities that I do to address stress? Well, the main areas that I have used and found can be helpful are exercise of various sorts, meditation, hypnotic triggers, food types, breathing techniques, appropriate sleep, music, time management practices, laughter and massage. There are many different ways of taking time out that others use, such as going for walks, playing golf, drinking at a bar, shopping, going fishing, taking a warm bath – not my personal preferences but they seem to be beneficial.

We've talked a lot about a whole variety of different types of exercise and there is undeniable evidence that this can help reduce stress. However, there are two very specific activities that we have not yet covered which I participate in very frequently.

The first is martial arts. In addition to all the physical benefits such as cardiovascular fitness, strength, speed and flexibility; there are innumerable other advantages that can be gained including self-control, empowerment, positive thinking, self esteem, assertiveness, improved attitude and determination, overcoming fears, advanced focus and concentration, superior reflexes and will power, increased self-confidence and discipline, added motivation and endurance, better co-ordination and posture, boosted energy and stamina, and so on. In fact it sounds like a whole book could be written in its own right!

Now superb stress relief can be obtained with martial arts because it includes stretching, breathing, relaxation, concentration, muscle tensioning & relaxing, balance, meditation and focussing. However, some of these could also be attributed to a few other sports or physical endeavours but what most martial arts have in addition, is engaging in more directly aggressive activities. So part of the training includes actually attacking your partner so that they can defend. It also includes kicking and punching bags or mitts. This can be extremely therapeutic and stress reducing and particularly helps reduce anger. Most martial arts also use a shout or 'kiai' when performing certain techniques. Such a form of controlled 'yelling' can also have enormous stress relief benefits!

Furthermore, one of the underlying subconscious factors of stress is fear. We all have experienced the fear of failing, of not being good enough, of not being liked, the fear of being confronted, and quite possibly the fear of being attacked. Martial Arts are a direct and overt approach to tackling fear. You learn to confront and overcome some very basic fears and this helps improve your responses to fear and stress in your everyday life.

Some of these added benefits are probably also found in related sports such as wrestling and boxing. All well and good, you might say but what about the inherent dangers in such a sport? Well, it appears that the risk of injury from martial arts is low compared to other sports. Most injuries are to the limbs and are usually quite mild such as bruises. When you have decided that you would like to join a martial arts class, you will need to checkout all the considerations I have already mentioned about joining a gym which is in the chapter on Weight Lifting Exercise. You can certainly watch a variety of classes first so as to give you a good idea of the demands of each discipline; but most important is to ensure that you attend an accredited school.

The second special activity is dancing. Many people do not realise how good a form of exercise this is. In fact, if you look on other forms of aerobic exercise as boring then you should definitely consider taking up dancing! Dancing is also pretty low-impact. Researchers at the Mayo Clinic maintain that social dancing provides many health benefits such as helping reduce stress, increasing energy, and improving strength, muscle tone, and coordination. Dancing can also burn as many calories as horse riding or walking. According to the National Heart, Lung, and Blood Institute (NHLBI) in the U.S.A., other benefits of dance are in lowering coronary heart disease risk, decreasing blood pressure, and managing weight. Another benefit of dancing is that the weight bearing movements can strengthen the bones of your legs and hips, which we all know is important as we get older. If all that wasn't enough, a study reported in the New England Journal of Medicine suggests ballroom dancing decreases the odds of suffering from dementia by 76%!

When you attend lessons or socials, you make exercise a fun and enjoyable event. Your "work out" takes place with pleasant music and you mix with other revellers who are in a good mood. What could be more fun and relaxing? Other general benefits include overcoming shyness, being able to dress nicely, improving your social life and meeting new friends, acquiring more poise, increasing self confidence, better co-ordination and posture, and boosting stamina. More importantly for this chapter, dancing is a perfect way to relax too because concentrating on dancing takes your mind away from the stressors of a typical day. You will probably also find that you will sleep better!

Regular (preferably daily) meditation is another very important part of a stress management regime. Unfortunately many of us feel that activities such as sitting in front of a TV are relaxing. In fact, research shows that being bombarded with ads, images, and sounds from TV is far from relaxing. Your mind is not quiet or calm or empty – all important for true relaxation. Moreover, TV viewing is a sedentary activity, and has been proven to be a significant factor in childhood obesity according to studies in Canada. Research into subjects' reactions to TV is disturbing – while watching TV, most of us report feeling relaxed and passive. What is surprising is that the sense of relaxation ends when the set is turned off, but the feelings of passivity and lowered alertness continue. Survey participants commonly reflected that television has somehow absorbed or sucked out their energy, leaving them depleted. They say they have more difficulty concentrating after viewing than before. In contrast, they rarely indicated such difficulty after reading, playing sports or engaging in hobbies where they reported improvements in mood. After watching TV, people's moods are often worse than before. Moreover, contrary to appearances, it seems that muscles do not tend to relax either when sitting in front of the TV.

Research has indicated that stimulating the hypothalamus gland in the brain by practising relaxation such as meditation helps to turn down the reactions to stress and causes a wide variety of beneficial physiological and biochemical changes that are the opposite of the stress response thus restoring our bodies' homeostatic balance and improving our disease resistance. In the next chapter, we will go into some techniques of meditation more deeply.

Many of us are reluctant to admit that we talk to ourselves in our minds. In reality, we all do this and indeed we would not be able to reason nor probably think at all without our internal self-talk. However, this mechanism can sometimes go seriously wrong and lead to mental illnesses such as schizophrenia. But even for the rest of us, our continual internal chatter can be detrimental to our general health if used incorrectly. For example, those with recurring symptoms of anxiety and nervous tension are usually barraged by a constant stream of negative self-talk. We need to replace these often critical and pessimistic statements with positive thoughts, declarations and messages. This is done by creating and frequently stating affirmations and we will address this in some depth in the next chapter. In particular, we can replace the negative views and feelings by more relaxing and stress reducing thoughts. We all need to work on worrying less and we can start by taking note of what Winston Churchill is believed to have said "When I look back on all these worries, I remember the story of the old man who said on his deathbed that he had had a lot of trouble in his life, most of which had never happened.". Another British Prime Minister (from the 19th century), Benjamin Disraeli said "Worry - It steals the bloom from the cheek and lightness from the pulse; it takes away the appetite, and turns the hair grey." There must be something about (British) politics!

By the way, there are certain things in our modern world that continuously bombard us with negative comments, images and statements that we can easily redress with just a little effort. One is the mobile (and even home) phone. It astounds me how some people allow this to intrude totally into their lives and dominate them. Quite frankly, I turn my mobile phone off continuously – when I'm eating, in the bathroom, in meetings, sleeping (yes, there are those who leave it on at night!) and so on. Other impositions include the TV and newspapers. The amount of negative, disturbing sensationalism is amazing and let's be honest, most of it is irrelevant. There are many of us who have benefited from the relief of turning off the TV and not buying newspapers!

I recall when I used to commute by train to work (not something I have done much of in my life!) and like most other passengers, I used to read the paper every morning. One day, near the end of my half hour journey, I happened to glance at the date on the paper – it was over a week old and I hadn't even noticed! It made me realise that the news from day to day was all the same, nothing much changed; same old doom and gloom; same irrelevant stories; same old propaganda ….

A very simple alternative is to listen to your favourite music; preferably uplifting, fun, happy, exciting, pleasurable music. Don't achieve this by turning on the radio – you'll still get assailed by negative news and boorish DJs! Put on your own favourite music. If it makes you get up and dance, even better – well perhaps not on the train! By the way, there are several studies that have shown that enjoyable music can help bring relief from pain of all sorts. So create your own collection of favourites and play them rather than listening to somebody else's selection.

So what else can we do to counteract this bombardment of negativity? Humour is frequently cited as a good tonic. There have been numerous studies and revelations about the healing power of comedy. The most commonly quoted is about a man who recovered from cancer by watching funny films and shows almost non-stop for weeks. How about creating your own humour library with your favourite cartoons, comedy albums, joke books, funny video films and humorous websites? However, there are a few rules about telling jokes to others – Avoid "put-downs" since it will just be a matter of time before you offend someone; Don't laugh at your own jokes; Know when to stop joking and be more serious because it can be very frustrating trying to communicate with someone who refuses to take you seriously. So don't forget – laugh and the world laughs with you but remember if you can stay calm while all around you is chaos then you probably haven't completely understood the seriousness of the situation!!

By the way, not only does laughter relieve stress but ironically many of the muscles we use to laugh are the ones that typically stay tensed up in our faces causing wrinkles. When we laugh then loosen them, we release that tension from our faces. It also appears to be good at protecting your heart according to the Center of Preventive Cardiology at the University of Maryland Medical Center. Researchers there found that subjects with heart disease were 40 percent less likely to laugh in humorous situations than those with healthy hearts! So remember, we don't stop laughing because we grow old; we grow old because we stop laughing.

One approach to get away from it all and wind down any current feelings of stress is to use breathing techniques. If I am feeling harassed or stressed, I frequently just stop and spend a few moments to take several slow deep breaths. Most of us tend to use our chests to breathe which is a habit we seem to have been taught by other adults – most children breath with their abdomen and this method is certainly recommended by the gurus. In particular, persons with asthma, a tight belt, a full stomach or those who are short of breath tend to resort to high breathing, way up in the chest. When encountering stress, one of our first responses is to hold the breath, or breathe very shallowly, so learning to correct this would be very beneficial. Most breathing techniques are grounded in yoga and are essentially a form of meditation. I must confess that I have no expertise in yoga but there are certainly many claims made about its efficacy in helping to relieve stress. I can make the same statement about Tai-Chi. There are many books, publications and classes where you can learn a variety of practices but one basic approach to beneficial breathing is to straighten up your posture then slowly (say to a count of 4) breathe in through the nose, starting with the very lower part of your lungs using your abdomen and gradually filling up to the top.

Pause for a count of 2 then gently exhale from the top of your lungs first, gradually down to the bottom. Wait for a count of 2-3 before inhaling again. The lower part of our lungs is seldom emptied sufficiently, and can accumulate air saturated with waste products; so after exhaling, when all the air seems to be out, push the stomach in slightly to expel any remaining. Only take a maximum of about six of these types of breaths as you might get a little dizzy due to hyperventilation, especially when starting out.

According to medical experts, such breathing techniques can be very beneficial to sufferers of phobias, anxiety or panic disorders. A variety of breathing and relaxation techniques have also been advocated by specialists (such as the Asthma Foundation of Queensland) to assist in the control of asthma. There is much evidence that it can also assist in stress-related heart conditions, insomnia and chronic pain. By the way, these breathing methods can be done standing up, sitting down normally, or wherever. You certainly do not have to learn some convoluted position like lotus to gain the benefits. Just try doing it in the car at traffic lights and see how much better you feel! Or consider it in a tense meeting or during a heated argument. To finish off this section on breathing, how about this quote that I came across from the Beatitudes (apparently as translated directly from the Bible in Aramaic) - "Blessed are they who are intimate with their Breath, for they shall receive the 'I Can' of the Universe."

We have all seen and personally experienced the effects of too little sleep; our concentration and effectiveness suffer, our energy levels decline and we get more stressed. Ironically the more stressed and anxious we become, the more difficult we find it to get to sleep and so it goes on in a vicious circle. A professor of neurology at the University of Minnesota Medical School has cautioned that sleep deprivation will diminish mental performance. Also work by a professor of medicine at the University of Chicago, found that metabolic and endocrine changes resulting from a significant sleep debt mimic many of the hallmarks of aging such as diabetes, hypertension, obesity, and memory loss. Studies by another Professor in the School of Medicine at Stanford University in the U.S.A., indicate that poor sleep can seriously alter the balance of hormones in your body. He concluded that this makes the sleep/wake cycle, also called the circadian rhythm, a good indicator to cancer prognosis.

So what can be done to help sleep better? The National Sleep Foundation and The Bellevue Hospital's Sleep Disorders Center in the U.S.A. offer several tips for helping us maximise the sleep we get during times of high stress and anxiety. These include: Don't expect to fall asleep immediately after hearing or watching disturbing news - stop listening to or watching news programs at least one hour before going to sleep. Engage in a relaxing, non-alerting activity at bedtime such as reading or listening to music. For some (not me personally!), soaking in a warm bath or hot tub can be helpful. Avoid activities that are mentally or physically stimulating. Do not eat or drink too much before bedtime. Only get into bed when you're tired - If you don't fall asleep within 15 minutes, get out of bed, go to another room and engage in a relaxing activity such as reading and only return to your bed when you're sleepy. Avoid nicotine, especially close to bedtime. Do not exercise within three hours of bedtime. Personally, three hours sounds excessive – I have frequently gone to bed within half an hour or so of energetic exercise and found that it actually helps me sleep.

Another technique is to write persistent thoughts and worries down in a notebook so as to get them out of your mind. Some pundits recommend keeping the same bedtime but I confess that I have never done this and never have much trouble sleeping. Certainly cutting back on caffeine and alcohol in the evening will probably help. Many imbibers find that if they drink alcohol to excess, they wake up in the middle of the night and cannot get back to sleep.

I certainly could not recommend taking sleeping pills. I took them once in my life and I have to say that partially waking up during the night and experiencing the total lack of control was not a pleasant feeling. Nor was the long lasting effect of drowsiness that continued well after getting up. It seems rather unfortunate that some persons counteract this by taking uppers in the morning and guess what – they have to take more sleeping pills the next night and so it goes on. If, like me, you don't want to wake up at the crack of dawn, you might consider investing in thick curtains on all the bedroom windows. I have frequently slept in rooms where there are Venetian blinds and I must say that their light exclusion abilities are rather poor! Another solution I have employed is to put on eye shades; the type you get given on aeroplanes. I find they help 'knock me out'; try them and see!

One related subject is napping. I have to say that I have practiced this habit most of my life whether on planes, in cars (while a passenger!), while waiting, wherever! Typically, I nap for half an hour or so and I have always woken up refreshed. Naps definitely can help make up for night-time loss. In a study of Japanese men, a mid-afternoon nap was shown to have positive effects on their daytime alertness. The 20-minute nap improved performance level and their self-confidence. Winston Churchill is rumoured to have recommended that "You must sleep some time between lunch and dinner, and no half-way measures.

Take off your clothes and get into bed…Don't think you'll be doing less work because you sleep during the day…You will be able to accomplish more."

We need to be aware that too much sleep can also have its own consequences. It was found by one University study that certain sleep characteristics such as continually sleeping for more than eight hours, regularly falling asleep during the day, and the tendency to snore influence the likelihood of having a stroke. Eight hours does seem to be a magic number - research continuously indicates that people are healthiest when they sleep about eight hours every night. Health problems are associated with both too much and too little sleep. But my experience indicates that it can be averaged - if some nights you don't get enough sleep, you can sleep extra the next night or two so that you're getting your required amount of sleep on average. In reality, other research has shown that there is no set amount of sleep everyone requires. It varies from person to person based on genetics, personality, diet, hormonal levels, and life demand.

Other research that I discovered many years ago indicated that we sleep in cycles of about one and a half hour durations. I therefore tend to organise my sleep as periods of 6 hours, seven and a half hours or nine hours. So if I am too late to get a full seven and a half hours, I will stay up a while and catch six hours. By the way, these numbers are sleep time, not time in bed which can be somewhat different for many persons. At the same time I also learnt some very powerful techniques for getting to sleep which are based on meditation. If you aren't aware of such things, you might like to practice the Progressive Muscle Relax and the Relaxation Response described in the chapter on Meditation. These are two basic methods that are very easy to perform.

One particular complication is sleep apnea (or spelt. apnoea), a disorder caused by muscles relaxing during sleep. It usually occurs in association with fat buildup or loss of muscle tone with aging. During an episode of obstructive apnoea, the windpipe collapses. This blocks the air flow while the sleeper struggles to breathe. The blood oxygen level falls and the brain responds by awakening the person. This cycle may be repeated hundreds of times a night and can be very detrimental to the brain. It may also lead to personality changes such as irritability or depression, and because it also deprives the person of oxygen, it can lead to a decline in mental functioning and an increased risk of stroke or heart attack. Loud snoring, frequent morning headaches, and excessive daytime sleepiness could be an indication of sleep apnoea. If you believe that you are suffering from it there are a few factors that you might be able to address such as

- avoid being overweight, quit smoking, eliminate alcohol in the evenings and particularly avoid getting drunk, remedy any allergies or respiratory infections, check the side effects of drugs such as sleeping pills or tranquilisers. If it doesn't improve then you might need to see a specialist who might recommend various equipment or surgery.

Other ways of helping to get to sleep are using self-hypnosis or other trigger mechanisms. Hypnosis is too detailed a subject to go into in this book but if you are interested there are many books and courses that address it. We use triggers frequently in life without giving them too much regard - for example, the classic 'tying a string around your finger' to jog your memory. There is also the famous response of Pavlov's dogs who after conditioning would salivate at the mere sounding of a bell. Perhaps certain smells or times of the day will initiate hunger in you. There are also many triggers that affect us sub-consciously – some might cause us to get stressed, afraid, depressed or better still, happy. Of course phobias are a typical form of trigger or anchor. Many elite athletes as well as prominent figures or performers have learnt to use triggers to induce a desired physical or more often, a mental response such as being focused, calm, confidant or motivated. This is particularly useful when they are about to perform or speak. There was a time when like many car drivers, I found it very hard to stay totally alert while driving. So I created a trigger that whenever I held a steering wheel, I would be 'wide awake and alert' – I have never felt drowsy since while driving. We can use this approach to create triggers to help us sleep and some of you probably do it without even knowing, such as those that find the waves on the seashore soporific, or the sound of a clock ticking makes them drowsy. There are others who only sleep if the radio or music is on and many of us sleep much better at home where we can hear common, though perhaps to others disturbing, noises like traffic or animals. As a form of hypnosis, you can also create other triggers such as clenching your hand, touching your fingers, taking a long slow breath, turning onto your side, repeating a special phrase and so on. Another methodology is to use imagery – in the same way that worrying thoughts can elicit stress responses, pleasurable thoughts can trigger feelings of well-being and relaxation. The choice of image is yours but it is preferable to use the same one every time for a given function. Think of it as watching a video in your head. With each viewing you feel more and more relaxed. This is positive feedback - your body learns to associate your mental picture with feeling better and therefore relaxes you. A natural progression is to use it to help you sleep.

Of course, one very pleasant way to relieve tension is to have a massage. There are many different types from a basic 'rub down', through Swedish to Shiatsu or Remedial. Massage works on the skin and the underlying muscles. The skin is in fact the largest organ of the human body and is packed with nerve endings. The main result of massage is to stimulate the blood supply in the area in question. With softer massage techniques this can be pleasurable and relaxing; with firmer types it can be rather painful but perhaps useful in addressing rather 'knotted' muscles. According to the Australian Association of Massage Therapists, modern studies have shown that it can be used to successfully treat a variety of disorders including general stress, anxiety, arthritis, back pain, muscle tension, headache and high blood pressure. It also generates improved skin tone and speeds the healing of soft tissue injuries. I have certainly found getting massaged to be very beneficial as a physical stress reliever and also to relax overworked muscles caused by heavy exercise such as gardening or home Do-It-Yourself jobs!

We have mentioned previously, various ways of massaging yourself such as your feet, scalp and neck in the shower. We also described some self-massages for the face. We often hold stress and tension in our temples that can lead to headaches. So rubbing that area can bring relief and then move down to the hinge of your jaw to massage your jaw muscles. It is quite easy to also relieve tension in your own shoulders and upper back as well as your neck. Many headaches are caused by tension of the sub-occipital muscles which are quite deep under the back of your skull. Many folk get tremendous relief from very firmly digging your fingers (or thumbs) into this area. I would recommend that you attend a massage course as I did many years ago – it has been quite rewarding using it to help others and also to understand how to benefit from it personally.

My final subject to discuss regarding stress is food. There are certain foodstuffs that research indicates can aggravate stress and facilitate its onset. Conversely, a stressed body can deplete itself of various nutrients which is then detrimental to health. For example, the stress response triggers the production of higher levels of the hormones adrenaline and cortisol. These are produced by all types of stress experienced, from emergency situations to slower-acting stresses (such as pressure at work or traffic jams). These stress hormones use up large amounts of vitamins B and C, magnesium and zinc, frequently leaving insufficient for the body's general use for them. This means that, for example, vitamin C and zinc may not be available for collagen production to keep skin clear and to make white blood cells to fend off infections; there are less B-vitamins for energy production and mental function; while depleted magnesium can increase the likelihood of headaches and raised blood pressure. Raised stress levels can also increase the amount of oxidation damage, which affects various body tissues, and constantly raised cortisol levels interfere with tissue repair. So what can be done to restore levels of these nutrients? Well, the now frequent cry of "At least five portions of fruit and vegetables daily" plus eat whole grains such as wholemeal bread, brown rice, whole-wheat pasta are certainly good advice.

We are frequently told that cutting down on excessive coffee drinking would be an effective part of managing stress. Also, bursts of sugar from sweetened drinks, pastries, snack-foods, candies (sweets, lollies), etc can make you feel more energetic in the short term. However your body might react to stabilize abnormally high sugar levels by releasing too much insulin. This causes a serious energy dip shortly after the sugar high. These variations can cause mood swings and eventually aggravate stress. Too much salt can raise your blood pressure and put your body under strain. So an important stress management tip would be to reduce your intake of refined sugar and salt. We shouldn't forget also that excess glucose (the result of sugar intake) is converted to fat and stored.

So that's a whole potpourri of approaches for you to consider with regard to controlling stress and in so doing, help keep you more youthful. Clearly you need to feel comfortable with whichever you choose so that they suit you as an individual. Work on some of these methods and let me know how they benefit you.

Review of Chapter 14

In this chapter we considered the many stressors and some of the possible ill-effects we can allow to happen as a result. Some of the approaches we weighed up to address stress included:

Special types of exercise such as dancing and martial arts

Meditation

Stress management techniques

Positive thinking and affirmations

Avoiding the impacts of continual bad news stories

Preventing frequent interruptions

Humour

Overcoming worry

Music

Breathing techniques

Sleep

Self-hypnosis and triggers

Massage

Foods

Chapter 15 - Meditation, Affirmations and Visualisation

As we have seen, knowing how to truly relax is an important asset for a long, healthy, youthful life and in the previous chapter we mentioned how powerful meditation is, particularly as preventative medicine. It can also be useful as a curative to address an immediate issue which has caused a stress- induced problem, however the preventive benefits of regularly meditating cannot be overstated. There are many sources of information about meditation techniques so we will only cover here a few of the different forms, as well as some approaches for getting into a meditative state. Incidentally, in addition to the relaxation benefits, you can also assist your creativity, memory (physical and mental), attitude, health, goal setting, stress levels and many other areas of your life. An additional tool that can be used here is visualisation and we will cover some aspects of that also. Some studies have clearly shown that meditators consistently have younger biological ages compared to their chronological age. Certainly in studies such as one reported in 1972 in the Scientific American (volume 226), it was shown to affect the human metabolism by lowering the biochemical by-products of stress, such as lactate; as well as decreasing heart rate and blood pressure. In the previous chapter we mentioned negative self-talk and how helpful it can be to replace these typically critical and pessimistic statements with positive affirmations. In this chapter we will look in more depth at how to use affirmations and provide some ready-to-use examples. Affirmations are even more powerful if recited while in a very relaxed state such as that induced by meditating. This is almost certainly because you are able to bypass your conscious mind and communicate directly with your sub-conscious.

There are hundreds of studies from around the world that have indicated the huge range of benefits that can be achieved by meditating. But perhaps as important are the positive reports from those who practice it. This is clearly something that anyone can learn and enjoy. Meditation undoubtedly originated in Eastern religions such as Vedic Hinduism. However, most western meditators today do not practice it as part of an organized religion. One creed well known for its reliance on meditation is Buddhism and they are quite active in teaching it. As Buddha apparently said “Meditation brings wisdom; lack of meditation leaves ignorance. Know well what leads you forward and what holds you back, and choose the path that leads to wisdom.” Some traditions recommend certain physical postures for meditation, particularly the various cross-legged postures, including the famed Lotus Position. However, none of these are necessary. What is important is simply to be in a fairly comfortable position such as sitting in a chair; I personally do not recommend learning while lying on the floor – this creates habits that make it difficult to use in normal situations. You can sit and meditate in almost any environment. Initially, you will probably want to find a quiet, perhaps darkened environment but once you are practiced, this is not needed. In fact once skilled, you can meditate anywhere, even with your eyes open and moving.

So what is meditation? It usually refers to a state in which the body is consciously relaxed and the mind is allowed to become calm and focused. This practice of contemplation and attention is often formalized into a specific routine such as using repetitive activities like deep breathing, humming or chanting which help induce the meditative state. I like to divide the approaches into two types – those that work on clearing the mind or Passive Meditation; and those where you are specifically using words or images to work on an outcome which I call Active Meditation. The frequency and length of meditation periods vary tremendously depending on the school of thought but twenty or thirty minutes is probably a typical duration.

The Mind-Body Medical Institute, which is affiliated with Harvard Hospital, reports that meditation generates many beneficial biochemical and physical changes in the body collectively referred to as the relaxation response. This includes changes in metabolism and brain chemistry, as well as a lowering of heart rate, breathing, pulse rate and blood pressure. They established that meditation techniques have a very real effect on reducing stress, inducing deep relaxation and controlling the fight-or-flight response. Meditation also causes changes in brain wave production as measured by an EEG machine. While in the normal waking state, the brain is primarily in the Beta range of frequencies (14 - 21 cycles per second). In a state of meditation, the brain tends to slow down to the Alpha range (7 - 14 cycles per second). One of the first researchers to study the effects of meditation on brainwave production was Jose Silva who founded the Silva Method. Silva theorized that in addition to stress relief, meditation could also be used for enhancing creativity and developing intuition. I attended a Silva Method course nearly 20 years ago and still use many of the tools today that I learnt there, including how to rapidly enter an alpha state of mind.

One thing that Silva noted was that there were certain activities where most of us naturally enter the alpha state such as in the shower and in the bathroom. We have already talked about how useful the shower is for carrying out head, feet, neck, back and shoulder massage. Since we are likely to be in alpha at this time, it could be very beneficial to use affirmations and visualisations and we will consider later which ones you might utilise. We also effectively move into this alpha state when we start to daydream. Often while in this apparent inattentiveness, we come up with all sorts of excellent ideas, solutions to problems and inventions. I'm sure there have been times when you have thought of some superb idea while daydreaming, only to have completely forgotten it later. Well, one solution that I have found is to use Memory Pegs to transfer ideas out of alpha and into beta (our everyday waking state). These will be covered in a later chapter on Memory.

Let's now look at some methods of attaining the alpha state. If you are beginner, you might find it helpful to find a relatively quiet, slightly darkened environment, with your eyes closed and to sit up straight in a very comfortable chair. You will probably find it best to have your feet flat on the floor with your hands placed loosely on your lap. The first is a progressive muscle tense & relax approach and is a very good way to learn.

Take a few slow, deep breaths and concentrate your attention on your feet. Scrunch up your toes and release them slowly. Lift your feet off the floor a bit and bend the balls of your feet towards your heels end then relax them as you let them come to rest on the floor again. Concentrate on tensing your calf muscles (this might be a bit hard for some of you) and then letting them go. Next work on feeling your thigh muscles tense up then relax. Pause for a moment to notice how heavy yet relaxed the whole length of both your legs are. Move to your buttocks and squeeze them tight before releasing them. Now pull in your abdomen and after you have let go, check to ensure that your breathing is taking place down there. Tense all the muscles in your back then gradually see to it that they all move into a calm state. Next sound out your chest muscles before moving up to your shoulders which you can pull back or move in a circular motion before allowing all the tension to release. Gradually move down your arms to your fingers; tensing and releasing and notice all the tension and worry flowing out of your finger-tips. Now set your attention to your neck and tighten up the muscles there before starting to feel your head floating off as you furrow your brow and let it go before scrunching up your face and releasing. Open your mouth wide and let it partially close. Observe how completely relaxed both eyes are and pass your attention gently down your whole body ensuring this same feeling is propagated throughout. Remain in this relaxed state for as long as you wish. As you become more practiced, you don't actually need to tense and release the muscles – you can simply focus your attention on each part of the body in turn (perhaps imagine feeling it getting warmer), slowly moving up (or down if you prefer) and you will attain the same levels of deep relaxation.

More advanced forms of this type of meditation can be used to work on health problems, pain and so on, especially if combined with visualisation and affirmations.

Another related technique for entering a meditative state is to simply concentrate on your breathing. I say 'simply' but there are many who will find it difficult to stay concentrated – certainly a good reason to persevere! Indeed, one of the reasons that we enter the meditative state is because we are focussing on a relatively mundane thing to the exclusion of others (such as worrying or distracting thoughts). So again, sitting calm and relaxed with your eyes closed, ensure you are breathing slowly and deeply using your abdomen and start to notice the air passing through your nose with each breath. Focus your attention on your inward breath as the air passes into your nose and fills your lungs, then there is a pause before you feel your lungs start to gently push the air out again and feel it pass through your nose. Just keep observing this and without realising it, you will find that you are totally relaxed and calm.

A different type of technique is to use a mantra. This is a sound or word or phrase which is repeated over and over; so as to block out other unnecessary thoughts. Transcendental Meditation is a famous form of meditation which became popular during the late 60s and 70s particularly when the Beatles took it up. Each meditator apparently uses a sound which has no meaning as such. I have found it very beneficial to use a word such as "calm" or "peace". In fact using "calm" as an immediate trigger in times of extreme stress is an approach I have used for many years. So, with the mantra approach, once again, sit comfortably and relaxed with your eyes closed. Concentrate on breathing slowly and deeply. Take an even deeper breath, hold it then force it out slightly as you say to yourself "calm". Repeat this a few times then return your breathing to a regular slow and deep breathing with your abdomen and each time you breathe out focus on the word "calm" and allow the feeling of "calm" to permeate your whole body. An alternative way is to count your breaths (if you find yourself at a point that you've forgotten where you are up to, this is excellent – it just means that you are in an alpha state, so just start again from 'one'). If there is a special word or sound that you prefer, or that has a calming influence or meaning to you, then use that.

A rather different approach to entering meditation is to focus on an object with your eyes open. This is a rather more advanced technique so if you are interested I will leave you to start with those methods above and then to find out more for yourself by reading up on the subject or better still by attending one of the numerous courses available. A variation of this is to visualise an object with your eyes closed, such as a red apple and keep seeing this throughout your meditation induction period. Another important type of specialised meditation is what I would describe as 'moving meditation' and includes such activities as martial arts (including not only karate or kung fu but also iado, archery etc), Tai Chi (which after all is derived from martial arts) and even formalised activities such as the tea ceremony, flower arranging, origami and many other ritualistic pursuits mainly from Japan. By the way, the techniques mentioned above with your eyes shut could also be used to help you sleep. One difficulty for beginners meditating is that they often tend to nod off because they are not used to being so relaxed! For this reason, most schools of meditation work on keeping you in a state of alpha but not to fall asleep. So on the one hand I hesitate to recommend using it for getting yourself to sleep but on the other hand, it does work well! Perhaps the best approach is to use one specific method for sleep and others for actually meditating. In fact over time, the sleep technique becomes a stronger and stronger trigger.

Once in a meditative state, you can decide whether you wish to continue in a passive mode or use the alpha state in a dynamic way. In most Eastern forms of meditation, the intention is to keep the mind clear of all thoughts. This is not as easy as it might sound. Inevitably most of us will wander off into thoughts of all sorts and various approaches are used to move these thoughts away and continue with a clear head. In many schools, you are taught to observe your thoughts so that they lose their relevance and become mere objects of contemplation. I will leave you to investigate this passive form elsewhere, if you are interested, but move on now to some types of dynamic meditation, in particular visualisation and affirmations.

Visualisation techniques are used by many successful individuals from athletes and actors to public speakers. You can use them to help set goals, work on your health, overcome allergies and phobias, or simply to help you relax more quickly and fully. The important thing about visualisation is to see in as much detail as possible, with full colour and clarity. Also, see yourself as if you are an observer of a scene and then additionally move into the scene and experience it as yourself. Here are some common types of visualisation which I certainly use and which you too can carry out once in the meditative state:

1. Special Place of Calm

Think of a place or location where you feel comfortable, happy and relaxed. For some this means by the coast or in a forest. For others perhaps it is a favourite building. These can be real or imagined. However, it is probably best if it is somewhere that you can feel comfortable being on your own. Now view this scene with as much detail and colour as you can. Then add any sounds and smells. Also feel things such as the sand or grass under foot, or the wind on your face. You can walk around your special place in your mind's eye or just lie there observing the calming activities. Use this place regularly, especially when you are feeling particularly stressed.

2. Shrinking Problems or Pain

Imagine the pain or problem being in front of you and surround it with a large bubble of whatever colour you choose - especially a colour that might have some significance here. Then slowly shrink the bubble and its contents in size. Continue shrinking it till it is very small. Then finally shrink it to nothing. A slight variant on this is to move the bubble further and further away from you until it is no longer visible.

3. General Health and Anti-aging

The basic approach is to visualise yourself inside your own body working on healing the affliction by various means; perhaps cleaning it, repairing it, replacing it, helping your immune system heal it, or whatever creative way you can think of or has meaning to you. With regards to some of the areas covered in this book, I frequently use visualisation to work on my scalp and hair especially while in the shower; on my eyes, waistline, muscles, facial skin, etc. while exercising; my teeth and gums while cleaning them and so on. Visualisation has been used by cancer sufferers with some incredibly successful results.

There has been a lot written about the benefits of positive thinking and we touched on it in the chapter on Mental Attitude. Here, we will spend some time addressing affirmations which can be thought of as an extension to positive thinking. A generally positive approach to the world is powerful in itself and helps prevent the continually negative thinking and attitude that many folk have, which in its worst forms can lead to depression and psychosomatic illnesses. Affirmations are very specific statements about issues that you have decided to address - studies have shown that using them can genuinely redress the way the mind responds to everyday situations. Strange as it may seem, the subconscious mind cannot easily distinguish between reality (whatever that actually means!) and strongly imagined, visualised or stated views about the world. After all, what is a memory? What is a worry about some future event (that may; or probably will not occur in reality)? You can just as easily cause your mouth to salivate by thinking about food as you can by looking at real food. So when you repeat certain statements about subjects, your mind can be fooled into accepting them. These are even more powerful if stated directly to the subconscious while in the alpha state, where the conscious mind can be bypassed somewhat.

Just a few of the areas that you might want to address with affirmations are – stress management, health issues, undesired habits, phobia removal, anger reduction, improving self-worth, weight control, hair growth, skin clearing, eyesight improvement, teeth & gum health, various body modifications, general mental well-being and quitting smoking. As with visualisation, affirmations are used by many very successful persons to help them in their endeavours. Take Muhammad Ali, who certainly knew what he wanted and seemingly quoted from Claude Bristol, a self-help author when he said that it's the repetition of affirmations that leads to belief. And once that belief becomes a deep conviction, things begin to happen.

Perhaps the best place to start with is some typical affirmations that I use while performing some of the everyday activities already described so far. So while massaging my scalp in the shower, I will repeat to myself (or even aloud) "my hair is growing strongly and vigorously" and "my hair is all dark brown in colour". While doing eye exercises, I might state "my eyesight is excellent; I can see perfectly at short distances and at long distances". While cleaning my teeth, I usually say (to myself!) "my teeth and gums are perfectly healthy and strong" and "my teeth are beautifully clean and white". While doing facial isometrics, I might repeat "my skin is totally smooth and clear" or "here I have plenty of cross-linked elastin and my skin is taught and smooth" and "my eyes look like I have slept perfectly every night of my life". While meditating in a deep state for health benefits, I will chant to myself such things as "my arteries are perfectly clean, clear and healthy", "my heart is strong and healthy" and "I am fit and well and perfectly healthy; physically and mentally". While working out in the gym I often repeat to myself "My abdomen is flat, taught, tight and firm" and "The fat has all burnt away from my midriff". I often say to myself "I am calm and relaxed". Even if you find it hard to believe that such statements could have any effect, you must at least acknowledge that saying these positive affirmations will prevent you from thinking your constant stream of damaging negative assertions.

Now you can create your own affirmations in your own words for things that are relevant to you. Here is a list of fairly general and commonly used types of affirmations which you might also find useful. The first is quite famous –

- Every day, in every way, I am getting better and better.
- I am a totally worthy person.
- I eat only healthy and nutritious food.

- I handle stress and tension very effectively.

- I always think positive thoughts that make me feel good about myself.

- My breathing is slow, deep and even.

- My muscles are heavy, comfortable and relaxed.

- I practice meditation daily and I enjoy it very much.

- I do regular exercise and it gives me great pleasure and results.

- I am full of energy and self-confidence.

- I cope very well during times of stress.

You can find no end of examples in books and the internet but do ensure that you only use ones that feel comfortable for you – there is no point in having a load of religious or New Age oriented ones if they are not in synch with your own personal attitudes and beliefs. Here are a few points that are recommended for creating affirmations that are worth noting in order to make them more powerful.

a) You will find that it works best to word your affirmation in the present tense, as if the result has already occurred. So avoid statements such as "I shall one day be happy again". This just reaffirms to your mind that you are not currently happy and moreover, "one day" may be a long time away.

b) Avoid negatives. Your mind hears the actual statement and the negative gets lost. So “I do not want to be unhappy and stressed” enters your mind as “I want to be unhappy and stressed”.

c) Use the first person “I”.

d) You will find it beneficial to repeat the same affirmation a few times.

e) Rather than a long rambling affirmation encompassing everything at once, use a few clear and concise affirmations. However, do not have a huge number; work on half a dozen maximum at one time.

f) Ensure that you have a strong desire and belief in your affirmations so that they will be far more successful.

g) Write your affirmations down – studies have shown that goals are much more likely to be achieved if they are put down in writing rather than just remembered in your head.

One word of warning about some of the subjects in this chapter – don’t be fooled into thinking that affirmations, visualisation, goal setting and so on are sufficient on there own. Many of them will have limited effect (apart from feeling good for a while) unless you also take massive action. It is no good just dreaming about the way you would like things to be, you have to do something about it. Just ‘putting it out into the universe' will not do a thing. Neither God nor the universe is obliged to take any notice of somebody who doesn't do anything to help themselves. As Epictetus the philosopher put it centuries ago "First say to yourself what you would be; and then do what you have to do." Please use these techniques and contact me to let me know how successful you have been.

Review of Chapter 15

Meditation and associated techniques allow practitioners to benefit from true relaxation so that stress levels are dramatically reduced and health is improved significantly. They can also assist in creativity, memory, attitude and goal setting.

Some of the meditational approaches described that you can practice include:

- Progressive muscle tense and relax.
- Progressive focus along your body.
- Concentration on breathing
- Repeating of a mantra
- Object focus (physical or mental)
- Moving meditation
- Mind clearing

As an adjunct to dynamic meditation, visualisation was discussed and you would do well to savour such techniques as:

- Special place of calm
- Shrinking problems or pain
- General health and anti-aging

Affirmations, the powerful extension to positive thinking was looked at and you will be considering using your own versions to assist in working on your hair, eyes, teeth, skin, fitness, health, calmness, phobias and so on. You might like to review some of the examples given of commonly used affirmations to incorporate into your own regime, bearing in mind the recommendations presented for creating them.

There is a well known saying about our bodies which is also true about our minds – 'use it or lose it'. We've already explored how important it is to continue exercising our bodies as we age so that it continues to function and be healthy. Well there are many persons who, as they age, stop learning new things, stop taxing their mind and generally let their brains fade away. The only thing some older folk seem to do with their mind is recall long ago memories. Is this a natural function of the aging brain or simply that they have nothing else to occupy their mind with? New information clearly indicates that contrary to past belief, the number of brain cells that we have are not fixed. It appears that no matter how old you are, you are still able to grow new brain cells. The important thing surely is to keep active mentally. There are many activities that you can participate in even if you feel that you have little time or money; or are unable to get out much. So let's consider a whole range of purely mental activities plus some that are more physical as well. There will be some that can be carried out at home and others for those that like to get out more. In addition we will touch on the difference between right and left brain functioning plus how you can keep and improve your memory.

There are some simple things able to invigorate the brain like doing crosswords, memory games or working on puzzles and games of various sorts; reading, particularly detective and historical novels or non-fiction; or perhaps keeping up with current affairs. These do not have to be expensive – most of these would be available at the local library! Perhaps better still would be to join socially with others and participate in discussion groups or debating societies. Furthermore there are bridge or chess clubs, card game groups and adult classes of all descriptions where you can engage in mental stimulation. All places where as Michel de Montaigne the French Renaissance writer put it – "it is good to rub and polish our brain against that of others." Perhaps for many it is time to learn about all that new-fangled technology and particularly computers and using the internet, which in itself is a huge repository of freely available learning experiences. Other ways of keeping on your toes (excuse the pun) are to learn dancing, Tai Chi, Martial Arts and similar activities where you are continuously learning new steps and patterns – a great way to stimulate your brain and body at the same time! I really enjoy the stimulation of attending workshops of various types and aim to learn a new skill every so often, such as a language, hypnotherapy, massage, drawing, reflexology, painting, acting, a dance style, and of course writing. When you take up any of these or other activities, I would be interested to hear of its success in keeping your mind active and youthful.

There is a lot of literature describing the difference between the right and left halves of the brain and how important it is to use both. Basically, this theory from the sixties suggests that the left brain hemisphere is considered to be mainly responsible for logical reasoning and daily functioning, whereas the right side is active during creative and artistic activities. It proposes that most of us seem to be left brain dominant so that when we tackle everyday problems, we rarely use creative thinking abilities. Studies seemed to show that less than ten percent of people use their right brain in these circumstances. So you can find a lot of training and descriptions of how to bring the right brain more into play. Meditation and visualisation seem to help tremendously, as does practicing artistic endeavours. Some apparently right brain activities which are exceptionally good for stretching your mind are drawing, painting, pottery, craft-work, sewing, knitting and needlework. These are also good for your finger dexterity so have the added advantage of helping fight against arthritis. Other recommendations are acting, singing, playing musical instruments and writing. Everybody has a tale to tell – perhaps write an autobiography to keep the edge on your mind and who knows you might come up with a best-seller!

More recent research using brain scanners shows this dual brain model to be rather simplistic. Two clinical neurologists, one from the UK and the other from Germany have concluded that the difference between the two brain hemispheres is more that they have varying styles of operating. The left brain appeared to focus on detail, while the right seems to concentrate on the broader background picture. Whatever the actual configuration, there is no doubt that many of the exercises designed to help us utilise more of our 'right brain' capabilities are still useful and certainly valid in improving our creativity and memory. Many of these techniques involved using imagination and visualization and what better personage than Albert Einstein to endorse such pursuits by apparently writing "Imagination is more important than knowledge. For knowledge is limited, whereas imagination embraces the entire world, stimulating progress, giving birth to evolution".

As one old guy said "My memory's not as sharp as it once was. Moreover, my memory's not as good as it used to be." Indeed many of us will find that as we get older, our memory seems to get worse. This seems to be true not only for things that have actually happened recently but perhaps even more irritating we can't find the right word to use in a sentence. It's there on the tip of our tongue but when once we were articulate with a strong vocabulary, suddenly we get lost for the correct words. This can happen to many who are younger too and I suspect that stress is the main culprit. However, there is much evidence to suggest that it can worsen with age if we allow it. I mentioned playing memory games above. There are any number of these and I recall as a teenage Boy Scout playing “Kim’s Game” which was mentioned by Rudyard Kipling in his book “Kim” and of course described by Baden-Powell in “Scouting for Boys”. Kim was being trained to work as a spy and this game was to improve his observation and memory. The facilitator collects about a dozen items and puts them out on a table. The participants have a certain amount of time (say 1 minute but as you get better, maybe reducing this to 10-20 seconds) to study the objects before they are covered up or removed. They are now asked to describe what they saw. The number of objects is actually very important because our short term memories can typically only recall 5-7 items. If we try to cram more items in, we tend to lose some of those already being held. Interestingly, it isn’t ‘first-in-first-out’ memory storage – we tend to remember the first few and the last few. There are various approaches to overcome this and Kim’s Game aims to improve concentration. Samuel Johnson the historic British author also captured it well when he observed that “The true art of memory is the art of attention.”

There are numerous publications on ways to improve your memory including how to remember the names of strangers you meet. Most of the techniques tend to use visualisation and the more advanced are based on creating a storyline which seems to be a common method used by those with a natural ability. One well known method that I have learnt and used for years is based on Memory Pegs. To cut a long story short, the principle is to associate a visualised item with each of the numbers 1 to 10 say. These are then your memory pegs which you will remember for life. A very simple set of these could be based on the nursery rhyme “This Old man, He Played One …..” When you have a number of items to remember, you ‘simply’ visualise each item in an amusing, full colour, active relationship with the next free memory peg. As I mentioned already, most of us find it hard to normally remember more than 5 to 7 items, so ten memory pegs is a great step forward and more advanced systems go to tens and hundreds of pegs with a bit of practice. In addition to just memorising things, I use my memory pegs for another rather special activity. I’m sure you all have had the experience of thinking up some fantastic creative idea or some perfect words for a speech or conversation while in a state of reverie, only to totally forget them later. Well to avoid these irritating situations, I use my memory pegs while in alpha to be able to recall things later while I am in the normal everyday beta state.

It seems that there are certain foods that can improve memory. For example, scientists at the University of Sydney put residents from a retirement village through a series of mental tests. They discovered that those who took vitamin C regularly scored higher. A U.S. journal reported in 1999 that testing in Sweden revealed that people with low levels of folic acid were more likely to score poorly in memory tests. In 1996, another American journal mentioned a study on 260 people over sixty five which reported that the top performers in a series of mental exercises were those who ate the most fruit and vegetables and consumed the least saturated fat. Many studies have also shown that missing breakfast reduces a person's performance at work (or school).

Review of Chapter 16

Having concluded that the best way to keep a well functioning mind is to actively use it, we got a taste of some activities worth pursuing such as:

- Working on crosswords and other puzzles and games.
- Reading, particularly detective, historical novels or non-fiction.
- Keeping up with current affairs.
- Joining discussion groups, debating societies, bridge or chess clubs, and adult classes.
- Using computers and the internet.
- Learning Tai Chi, martial arts and dancing.

In getting a feel for the difference between right and left brain functioning we considered a range of other involvements including drawing, painting, pottery, craft-work, sewing, knitting and needlework as well as acting, singing, playing musical instruments and writing.

While touching on ways to keep and improve memory the following tools were described for you to practice:

- Kim's Game
- Memory Pegs

Certain foods that potentially improve your memory were mentioned.

Chapter 17 - Menopause and Andropause

There is one major occurrence in the life of a woman that can seriously impact on how she appears to age and that is the onset of menopause. Now males, please do not skip this section – it is a subject that has significant importance to your relationships with women. Moreover, in a few paragraphs later I will be addressing andropause which is a condition in men that causes similar symptoms.

There are huge amounts of information available to assist females in understanding about menopause and I am certainly no expert so I will only touch on the subject here. It is a normal occurrence in a woman's life which typically happens between the late 40s and early 50s. Normally it is due to the ovaries having run out of functioning eggs so the periods (or menses) cease. This is accompanied by substantial hormonal changes and especially with a reduction in oestrogen. Some of the almost immediate consequences include skin and hair deterioration, weight gain, mood swings, loss of energy, the infamous hot flushes and impacts on sex life. Interestingly for some women with a very optimistic attitude, the fact that birth control will no longer be a concern can lead to an invigorated sex drive – sounds like a very positive approach! On the other hand, the lowered sex drive is due to the ovaries producing less testosterone, the hormone that conventional wisdom associates with masculinity. More longer term issues that need to be considered include osteoporosis and heart disease.

Although menopause is unavoidable, you need to be aware that women who smoke tend to experience it around two years earlier than non-smokers. It is also possible that it may have been brought on early as a result of chemotherapy or ovary removal. This is known as medical or surgical menopause.

So what are the measures that you can consider to deal with the impacts of menopause? Well in a nutshell, it seems that many of the areas addressed in this book will already have a very positive result. For instance, general exercise will be quite therapeutic in terms of controlling weight, rebuilding bones, improving sleep, strengthening your heart, helping your skin glow, lessening hot flushes, increasing energy and boosting sex drive. I'm sure you'll agree that this is an impressive list of benefits and all achieved naturally with no side effects! So, for example, we have already discussed how resistance training (which includes not only weight training but also walking and dancing) can help slow bone loss and how aerobic exercise is excellent for improving cardiovascular health and general wellbeing.

If you're less physically active now than when you were younger, but consume the same number of calories, the result is likely to be weight gain. As people age, their metabolic rate often slows, so they need less fuel to maintain their normal weight. But studies show that the trend is the same for women and men, so it can't simply be blamed on menopause. However, menopause does seem to exacerbate this, so you will need to seriously consider reducing your calorie intake. This does not mean going on a diet but a permanent change in your previous lifetime's eating habits. More specifically, you might consider including high fibre, low fat foods that are rich in calcium and phytoestrogens. We have already reviewed how the consumption of calcium can improve your bones. But what is an adequate amount for women after menopause? Experts suggest that around 1,000mg a day is probably necessary. To assist in the absorption of calcium you should also ensure you have sufficient Vitamin D. As previously mentioned, safe sun exposure is the most natural way to achieve this. Phytoestrogens are compounds that occur naturally in plants and are similar to the hormone oestrogen so they are considered beneficial in relieving some menopausal symptoms. Useful foods here include soy and linseed.

Hot flushes may be triggered by such things as alcohol, caffeine, smoking, spicy food, or even hot baths or a generally hot environment. So keep note of these potential aggravators. In particular, many specialists in menopause propose that increased levels of caffeine can worsen not only hot flushes but also insomnia and night sweats. Unfortunately, it can also increase the risk of osteoporosis. According to several surveys, stressful situations are perhaps the biggest cause of hot flushes. We have a whole chapter concerned with stress control and you might like to review this since stress can also hinder the proper functioning of the adrenal glands and these assist in the production of oestrogen after menopause.

Following menopause some women feel that they are not so mentally alert and their memories get fuzzy. We have already addressed how retaining a good memory can be very dependent on mental conditioning so that the more regularly you exercise your brain, the better it will perform. So keep learning new things and practice memorising items such as names, birthdays and telephone numbers.

If you experience moderate or worse symptoms, your doctor might well recommend HRT (hormone replacement therapy). It seems to be an effective short-term treatment for menopausal symptoms and there has been considerable experience and studies to understand its benefits and side-effects.

By the time men reach the age of 40 to 55, many can experience a phenomenon similar to the female menopause, called andropause (sometimes called male menopause, though this term is very misleading and strictly inappropriate since men do not have menses!). Unlike women, they don't have a clear-cut event such as the cessation of menstruation; however, it is also precipitated by a drop in hormone levels. Whereas oestrogen is the hormone more relevant to females, testosterone is implicated here for males. More specifically, andropause is associated with low bioavailable testosterone levels. Every man experiences a decline over time but some men's levels dip lower than others. Whereas women have a very marked drop (up to 90 percent) in their oestrogen levels during the time of menopause, men have a more gradual decay in their testosterone levels. The symptoms include fatigue; weight gain; a loss of energy and sex drive; as well as changes in attitudes and moods. Certain health matters seem to contribute to its onset such as infections, medications, injuries and surgery.

For many men, it is probable that it can be avoided by addressing factors such as obesity, attitude, alcohol and stress. It will probably come as no surprise to you when I say that, as for menopause, all of the natural strategies necessary for tackling andropause are already contained in this book. So your lifestyle needs to incorporate approaches such as regular exercise, stress control, optimal diet, the reduction of alcohol intake (especially beer) and the elimination of tobacco.

Hormone replacement therapy for men is a far more controversial subject than for women. There are growing numbers of specialists who are proponents of such interventions because they have witnessed significant improvements in some men. However, there is little data yet on potential long term effects. Rather than the injections, creams, patches or pellets (inserted under the skin), a more natural way to boost testosterone might be with the herb Tribulus terrestris. Apparently this has been used for a long time to restore testosterone levels in Asia. It was reintroduced to the western world by East German athletes particularly at the Olympics. It is claimed to have both an aphrodisiac and a male performance enhancing effect. In addition to testosterone, another important hormone for male health and masculinity is DHEA which is also getting much publicity as a supplement.

There is another phrase that you might have heard - Irritable Male Syndrome! Its existence is strongly disputed by many experts in the field, especially the use of the term 'Syndrome'. Many of the symptoms are similar to andropause (which, as we have discovered, is itself controversial) but the emphasis is more on moods such as irritability, anger, impatience and even depression. The magic cure, as for andropause is claimed to be testosterone replacement therapy.

Review of Chapter 17

Menopause and andropause are caused basically by the naturally occurring reduction of sex hormones in the body. Many of the resulting symptoms can be alleviated by carrying out the recommendations already recommended in this book including:

Perform sufficient, appropriate exercise.

Modify your eating habits.

Practice stress management.

Reduce alcohol and caffeine intakes.

Stop smoking.

Keep your mind and memory active.

Chapter 18 - Food and Drink

I've already spoken at some length about food and diet in the chapter on the Abdomen and Waist but that was specifically concerned with keeping trim. In this chapter we will address food and drink more in respect to longevity and general good health. So we will need to consider the benefits, dangers, half-truths and in some cases downright lies about subjects as diverse as fish, processed meat, preservatives, hormones, fat, sugar, salt, artificial sweeteners, fresh fruit, supplements and the interesting discussion about just eating less. However, if we are taking care to eat food that keeps us healthy then we won't be like the woman who admitted that most of the items in her shopping cart were labelled "For fast relief"!

Compared to only a few decades ago, it is extraordinary how little food in our shops today is truly fresh. The mere fact that we only need to go food shopping once a week (or in some cases once a month!) is an absolute indication that the food is not fresh and is probably full of preservatives. I remember one day in January looking at a sealed plastic bag containing what was proudly declared to be "Fresh Noodles". It had a use-by date of mid April. This means that I could buy this product in April and it would still have been declared as 'fresh' when it would be at least three months old! The food processing industry has a lot to answer for with regards to the way that our food is manipulated and some would say filled with harmful chemicals. This ranges from the crude waxing of fruit to make it look appealingly shiny (or so the food industry believes) to pumping chickens, cows and other animals with damaging (to humans) hormones. I can remember when a delicatessen was a place where you could buy delicacies. Nowadays it seems to be where you buy pressed cardboard called processed meats. It looks and tastes as much like meat as instant coffee tastes like real coffee! The anaemic white gunge is laughingly called chicken. Once you used to buy ham cut off the bone; nowadays, it's a perfectly circular or even square piece of flattened pink stuff! Even so, the manufacturers still have the gall to call one version of it 'ham off the bone'! Another strange occurrence over the past few years has been the replacement of natural squeezed orange juice with a beverage manufactured from concentrate. Presumably it is cheaper in some way for a far away place with cheap labour to condense the juice, ship it to a local factory and then for water to be added. Goodness knows what affect this has on the natural attributes of fresh juice though frequently the factory adds vitamin C back in again. If you travel a lot internationally, where once you could rely on fruit juice being relatively safe to drink, nowadays it is made from concentrate with the local water added – just the thing you were trying to avoid!

If you look at the ingredients in foodstuff, you see more numbers representing the additives and preservatives than you do actual ingredients. I'm convinced that the extraordinary huge numbers of so-called food allergies that have broken out over the last decade or so are simply reactions to additives, especially preservatives and certainly studies have shown how they are making children in particular hyper-active and adults lethargic. So, the message here sounds simple – look at the contents lists and avoid those that are full of additives. Unfortunately, this is often easier said than done! Many items are starting to declare 'no preservatives, no added sugar, no artificial colours or flavours' and so on. So I certainly tend towards these but you still need to be careful about cynical marketing. For example, we all know that too much sugar is not healthy for us and so companies make declarations such as 'no added sugar' when what it means is no added cane sugar – it will probably be sweetened with corn syrup or some other 'sugar-tose'. Some processors use the term 'no artificial sweeteners' because apple juice, honey, molasses, fructose and even sugar from cane or beet is strictly speaking 'non-artificial'. Don't forget that the body doesn't really know the difference between sugars once it is digested. The important question is – how much sugar is there in the item and if it is anything over about 15% then you probably need to be wondering about its appropriateness. Even claims that honey is a healthy, natural sweetener need to be questioned. Nobody is doubting that honey might have some health benefits but the actual sugar in it is no different to sugar in 'natural' sugar-cane once the body has turned it to glucose!

So to avoid excessive sugar, the industry has come up with various artificial sweeteners and we are all jumping on the bandwagon. Saccharine was one of the first but some trials linked it with increases in certain cancers so it went out of fashion. Now there is aspartame which is in products like Nutra-sweet. This contains phenylalanine, an amino acid. There is a lot of controversy and dispute about whether there are dangers and side effects of aspartame. Ironically there are totally different studies that indicate that there are certain positive benefits of phenylalanine including its use as a 'smart-drug' (causing an increase in mental alertness). There are many who seem to crave sweetness but this is probably a form of habit which can be broken. There are various alternative flavourings that you could consider instead of sugar such as nutmeg or cinnamon or even throwing in some chopped fruit. One of the biggest culprits in terms of sugar loading seems to be so called soft drinks (a clever example of misleading marketing). Children especially can get caught out by these. It would be much healthier for them to drink unsweetened natural fruit juice mixed with plain or sparkling water.

Avoiding too much fat is another beneficial eating habit but once again, be careful of product labelling such as 'low-fat'. Just check the ingredients to ensure that they haven't simply added sugar instead – I remember being appalled to find that 'low-fat' biscuits or cookies had well over 50% sugar in them. Guess what the body converts excess sugar to – body fat! The original low-fat proposals turned out to be far too simplistic when it was discovered that there were many different types of fats and that some of them are actually beneficial to your health. Moreover, studies realised that products like margarine, which were aimed at avoiding so called bad animal fats were actually far worse because they contain an artificially created fat (called trans fat) that increased cancer risk! Actually, I was astonished the other day to read the ingredients list in a margarine to discover that the first item (therefore the biggest quantity) was animal fat! So, by all means keep your fat intake low but don't forget the health benefits of foods like avocado, peanuts, olive oil and canola oil which contain mono-unsaturated fats. Also nuts, which have a fair amount of fat in them contain mainly unsaturated fats which have many benefits. Research has shown that nuts also contain a range of other very healthy ingredients. Almonds in particular have been shown to increase your chances of living longer, as does eating an amount of dark chocolate (another item containing a fair amount of fat)! Hurray – the news isn't all bad! Except that sadly I have a suspicion that the age old concern that chocolate causes pimples or acne might be true. As previously mentioned, I rarely eat candy bars or chocolate but when I saw the reports about the benefits to your heart of eating dark chocolate, I started partaking! Unfortunately, within a few weeks I had a rash of pimples which took some months to clear up (after I stopped my indulgence and got plenty of sun!). Now when I researched this, there seems to be no scientific evidence that chocolate has this effect. So what is the experience of you readers?

The real good news story with regards to eating fats is fish. Cold water fish such as sardines, mackerel, tuna, trout, herrings and salmon are high in omega-3 fatty acids. These have a whole range of benefits. Not only do they increase your chances of living to a ripe old age by combating the classic killers of heart disease and cancer but it also seems to help ease the swelling and pain of rheumatoid arthritis! One University study over 12 years ago found that men have a 25 percent less chance of developing prostate cancer by eating fish three times a week. Alzheimer's disease and dementia were also shown to be reduced by a U.S. Government 2005 analysis. As it happens, trials of fish oil supplements showed similar results as eating the real thing!

So we all know that the western diet is too full of sugars and fats which appear to be the main culprits responsible for the proliferation of diseases which kill us with cancers and heart failures. Included in this list is also excess salt which is used as a 'natural' preservative but more recently as an over-used flavour enhancer. Interestingly the dangers of MSG (monosodium glutamate) seem to be clear to all but there are large numbers of consumers who apparently ignore the problems caused by ingesting too much salt. Perhaps part of the reason is that it is often 'hidden' in processed foods such as cereals, cakes, pastries and meats. As a guide, anything that has a sodium content higher than 500 mg should be viewed with suspicion, especially as the daily recommended maximum is 2,300 mg. There have been many studies showing that the main health issues with salt are that too much can increase blood pressure and hasten heart attacks.

One major way that we end up partaking of too much of these items is through unhealthy snacking. The supermarket shelves are full of chips, candy bars, biscuits, crisps, cookies and a multitude of packets of manufactured 'goodies' (sadly they are not very 'good' for us!). It would be well worth your while to consider substituting these products with healthier choices. So try raw vegetables or low-fat cheese instead of cookies, biscuits, sweets, lollies and candy; try wholegrain crackers instead of cookies or biscuits. One serious rule to note here is that 'supersizing' is NOT a bargain!! Consider the dangers of being tempted to pay a bit more money for a lot more fat, sugar and salt.

What other things should you consider limiting in your diet? Well you must be aware of the overwhelming evidence about drinking excessive alcohol. As you know, it's right up there with too much sugar, salt and fat in terms of increasing your risk of dying early of a fatal disease (not just heart problems and cancer but also liver damage), as well as reducing your youthfulness and fitness. In fact it also seems that too much alcohol causes dehydration which might cause fine lines on your skin. Having said this, we mustn't ignore other research which shows very clearly that certain alcohol, especially red wine can be quite beneficial to your heart! But as always it is a matter of moderation – I believe the recommended amount is no more than two glasses a day. The recuperative powers of wine when used in moderation were already being lauded thousands of years ago by Hippocrates who noted "Wine is fit for man in a wonderful way, provided it is taken with good sense by the sick as well as the healthy".

While reviewing liquids, what about water? There is an amazing amount of hype at the moment about how apparently important it is to drink large quantities of water – at least 8 glasses a day the pundits suggest. Well, I have never drunk such an amount of water and I am never dehydrated as the self-professed experts predict. Nor am I poisoned by my own (perfectly capable) kidneys. Let's face it, if my body had insufficient water, it wouldn't let me urinate and I have no problems performing this activity! I have to say that I am rather bemused by the sight of those wandering around clasping a huge plastic drinking bottle all day as if it was life and death – and sadly if you've ever attended certain health seminars, this is the principal message that seems to be proposed. So I did some searching and try as I might, I was unable to find any evidence whatsoever for this apparent wisdom of drinking so much water. Perhaps it would be sceptical of me to suggest that all of the arguments in favour have been created by the powerful soft drinks industry. It is extraordinary how much the sales of bottled water have risen over the last decade into the billions of dollars (the same period over which all these recommendations have been appearing!). Perhaps not so surprising after all, when you realise that the marketing and PR by these same companies has persuaded huge numbers to start drinking coloured water full of salts and sugars calling them sports drinks; just the ingredients that the medical fraternity has been suggesting we avoid! Now of course while you are exercising, it is important to replace fluid loss, especially if the environment is warm.

Well, enough said about things to avoid; what about those that are beneficial for keeping youthful and even rejuvenation? I've already mentioned the benefits of fruit for helping to keep slim. They contain piles of vitamins, minerals and trace elements. They are low in calories (kilojoules) and are a natural laxative. Similar good things can be said about fresh vegetables. From my perspective, you can never eat too much of either and they are the staples of my diet. With regards to vegetables, apparently mushrooms (which I always include in my shopping) rate as number one for such benefits as riboflavin, niacin, pantothenic acid and biotin as well as a source of several other valuable items. Other foods with claims to fame include: Blueberries and other berries like raspberries, blackberries and strawberries are rich in antioxidants. Walnuts have several nutritional goodies such as omega-3's, fibre and the antioxidant vitamin E. Tomatoes are one of the best sources of lycopene, an antioxidant that apparently protects against prostate cancer in men. I notice a lot of attention being paid to eating raw foods as a means of staying healthy and even rejuvenating and I must confess that more and more of my diet is raw fruit and nuts with some raw vegetables and others that I cook for only a short time. It is often difficult for us to point to a specific food item or constituent as definitely being responsible for a health, vigour or youthful property; however, there is no doubt that when I changed to a mainly fruit diet I definitely felt better than I had ever experienced before. Do you have any such instances that you can share?

Several previous chapters have mentioned foods that are beneficial such as that dealing with memory and the one referencing eyes. Some of you might be surprised to learn of a study of more than 90,000 Japanese residents which was published in a cancer journal. It showed that those who drank one or two cups of coffee daily had half the risk of liver cancer than those who did not. On the other hand, nobody is likely to be surprised at studies indicating that some foods we consume can upset our skin. Researchers at an Australian university, have been studying how the food we eat can influence how our skin is affected by the environment. Hundreds of elderly people in several countries participated as part of the international study. Some of their conclusions were that the following foods may contribute to producing wrinkles - full fat milk, red meat, potatoes, soft drinks and cordials, cakes and pastries. On the other hand those that may help prevent wrinkles included – eggs, yogurt, vegetables, nuts, olives, fruit, tea and water as well as mono-saturated fats, vitamin C and retinol (Vitamin A), calcium, phosphorus, magnesium, iron and zinc.

The age old advice is to eat everything in moderation. It has certainly been known for a long time and was probably first stated by Hippocrates, the ancient Greek physician as "If we could give every individual the right amount of nourishment and exercise, not too little and not too much, we would have found the safest way to health." Ironically, one of the most proven methods of prolonging your life is to eat less. It has been shown in every investigation with animals of many types such as rats, rabbits, dogs, mice, guinea pigs, and even fruit flies. They all lived about one third longer when they were fed less. But more importantly, they also behaved and looked younger. Two researchers at the University of Washington, Seattle discovered that the restriction of food slows the rate of cell division, which effectively slows aging.

There have been a number of theories of aging, such as free radical damage, collagen loss or glycosylation. But these have later been shown to be effects of aging not the cause. Scientists' understanding of the aging process was dramatically updated by an article published in 1990. Leonard Hayflick had already discovered that cells divide about 80 times and then stop. But the new finding explained why our cells stop dividing. The discovery was that there is an inbuilt mechanism that limits the number of times a cell can divide. It is controlled by a part of DNA called a telomere. In fact, the age of a cell can be measured by its 'telomeric length' and as the telomere shortens with each division, the cell programmes its own death. Other researchers have found that high levels of homocysteine (an amino acid) in the blood can triple the amount of telomere length lost when a cell divides. So those bodies are aging more quickly. It is therefore no surprise that high levels of this substance are related to heart disease, Alzheimer's disease, Parkinson's disease, impotence and other common degenerative diseases of aging. A doctor can measure homocysteine with a blood test and apparently it can be corrected with some basic supplements; in particular Vitamin C, Vitamin B12, Folic Acid, Vitamin B6, Riboflavin (Vitamin B2) and trimethylglycine.

So what about supplementation? Many cynics have stated that taking vitamins is just an expensive way to create coloured urine! Well I have to say that I agree with the opposing view that if you are living a full active life then it is quite likely that you are not always ingesting sufficient of everything you need so it is a good insurance policy to take a multivitamin tablet regularly. Even if you are eating an apparently very healthy diet, sometimes the soil might be deficient in certain important minerals. Certainly, in countries like Australia, this is true. There is a particular concern right now about the lack of iodine. For many years iodine has been an additive to table salt since it has been a common deficiency in many places around the world. But guess what? With all the negative press about the dangers of salt, many of us are no longer getting sufficient iodine!

There have been all sorts of claims by suppliers about their supplements and no doubt many of them are true such as Vitamin C being necessary for the formation of collagen and zinc assisting in tissue repair. However, there is also frequently a lack of thoroughness in the presenting of research data. So for example, a study might be referenced which shows that a certain compound can be beneficial. However, it may have failed to mention that it was an extremely large amount that needed to be taken over a certain period of time in order to obtain the benefits.

Theories about Vitamin C prolonging life were not accepted by the rest of the scientific community until anti-oxidants were discovered in the 1980s. This is when the whole theory of anti-oxidants including Vitamin C protecting against free radicals was formed. The aging effect of free radicals is not so much caused by cell damage but by oxidative damage to the telomeres (which we have already come across above). Japanese research reported in 1998 showed that high levels of Vitamin C could slow the loss of telomeres by as much as 60%. Unfortunately the amount of Vitamin C used to achieve this was at least 500mg twice a day – far more than a normal vitamin tablet!

Review of Chapter 18

After noting how poor the quality of many foods are, this chapter considered a few of the nasty additives and preservatives that today's food processing companies put into our food and some of the resulting potential ill-effects. It also reviewed some of the studies that have shown us why we should be careful not to partake of too much alcohol, fat, sugar and salt amongst other items. Several warnings were proffered about how manufacturers try to fool us with wording on packaging. There was even a challenge to the veracity of the commonly held belief that we should drink large quantities of water. Thankfully, it was rather better news about the benefits of eating fish, avocado, nuts and even dark chocolate! In fact red wine also got a good rap (in moderation!). The real stars were of course fruit and vegetables. Although pill-popping is not a general recommendation in this book, the benefits of several supplements were mentioned. Regardless of all the preceding information, several studies have shown that perhaps the most significant impact on slowing aging is simply to eat less!

You can probably guess that this chapter will not be condoning the habits of cigarette, alcohol or drug abuse. I'll try hard not to lecture but since I do not smoke or take drugs and rarely drink alcohol, I believe this is an important part of the overall picture of looking more youthful.

Well I'm sure that those of you who smoke do not need me to go through the whole list of health problems that are caused by your habit. Sadly, I have known smokers personally, who over periods typically of a couple of decades or sometimes much less time have deteriorated dramatically in health. Gradually their whole body has succumbed; from stomach ulcers and chest complaints; to serious thyroid, liver and digestive problems; and finally to a horrid destruction by cancer and death. As we all know, even so called "passive smoking" can be very deleterious – far worse than a French novelist even realised when she admitted "My smoking might be bothering you, but it's killing me". As already mentioned in this book, it is not easy for smokers to look young although they may never live long enough to look old! Apart from the general ill health, coughing, stained fingers, bad teeth and so on, there is the inevitable horrid smell. The tobacco industry has a lot to answer for, from apparently hiding damaging research, to targeting children and third world countries to a whole range of cynical advertising including the pretence that so called 'lite' cigarettes are somehow healthy. But with the combination of huge profits allowing money to talk; enormous lobbying; lucrative advertising and marketing contracts; and vast tax revenues, our elected governments do not seem to have done much to protect us. It seems extraordinary that within living memory, most armed forces supplied cigarettes as part of their remuneration. In their hypocrisy, governments all over the world are reluctant to lose the enormous revenues that they receive. But this is not a new phenomenon. In the eighteen hundreds, Napoleon III, the French Emperor, when asked to ban smoking (whose evils have been recognised since Sir Walter Raleigh first brought it from the New World) retorted "This vice brings in one hundred million francs in taxes every year. I will certainly forbid it at once - as soon as you can name a virtue that brings in as much revenue"

I guess it is easy to tell that I am a non-smoker (or perhaps a reformed smoker). In fact, I gave up cigarette smoking when I was 11 years old! In the fifties it was possible for a 7 year old to go and buy cigarettes – even single ones! I was in the Boy Scouts and I remember reading "Scouting For Boys" by the founder Baden-Powell. His chapter on the ill effects of cigarettes was enough for me to vow that I would quit.

Considering that he wrote this book in the early 1900s and that he was a military man, he was clearly far-sighted in his views. Luckily the chapter on sex (something to do with the sap rising in spring as I recall!) was incomprehensible, so I didn't have to give that up before I started! While I'm on a hobby-horse about the negatives of smoking, I should mention how much non-smokers cannot believe the selfish, anti-social attitude of most smokers in terms of littering, causing of fires and the danger to cyclists and soft-top cars when lighted cigarettes are thoughtlessly disposed of. This is all on top of the cost to society due to damage, health services and lost productivity.

I'm sure it would be disputed vehemently by those in denial but it seems to me that cigarette smoking is frequently the first step towards stronger drug taking – do you know anybody on drugs who hasn't been (or probably still is) a smoker? Ironically the list of health problems caused by drugs doesn't seem to be as long as for cigarettes. This is presumably because most drug addicts die very young! Marijuana, which so many have tried to convince themselves was harmless, in fact seems to have plenty of long term effects. While I was growing up, there were plenty of drugs available from amphetamines to cocaine and LSD but luckily I couldn't afford it! Perhaps more importantly, I didn't find it very appealing – I wanted to stay in control of my life. While I was at university, I saw some of the devastation caused by drug taking. I vividly remember a student we dubbed the bread pudding boy – as a cheap meal, I used to make bread pudding and one night this guy really tucked in with relish as it was the only thing he'd eaten all week. Having become a heroin addict within a few months of starting university, he was emaciated, weak, could barely converse, was incomprehensible when he did talk, certainly couldn't study and dropped out of Uni a few months later. I heard that he dropped out of life a year or so after that!

I have just been watching the film 'Walk the Line' about country singer Johnnie Cash. It reminded me somewhat of similar films like the story of the Doors – good films overall but some of the scenes were pretty sad and rather pathetic. Some of the side effects (perhaps it would be more correct to say, the real effects) of drugs were seen in these films. The list is enormous and depending on the actual concoction ranges from a dry mouth, raised blood pressure, reduced libido, kidney disorder, restlessness, impaired short-term memory, nausea and ineffectual body coordination, through anxiety, panic and confusion, leading to depression, paranoia and suicidal urges. Very large doses can cause convulsions, coma and brain haemorrhage or even death through heart or respiratory failure An overdose can cause rapid heartbeat, heart failure, shortness of breath, unconsciousness, coma and of course death. Common side effects after coming down from drugs include depression; tiredness; and feeling irritable, restless, dizzy and anxious. Holland, which has had very liberal laws (i.e. almost none!) regarding drug use, is now facing significant social issues with those hard drug addicts who have managed to survive. As they grow older, they are facing in their forties the sorts of problems normally experienced in very old age - they are forgetful, neglect themselves, suffer from insomnia and live in isolation. Many users are in blind denial of the long-term effects but it doesn't take a scientific study to observe the impact on ex pop stars and actors who have clearly abused their bodies over the years. As one of the more honest famous celebrities, Billy Holiday (jazz singer) allegedly said "Dope never helped anybody sing better or play music better or do anything better. All dope can do for you is kill you – and kill you the long, slow, hard way." And she would have known. An even more famous pop musician put it this way 'That's all drugs and alcohol do, they cut off your emotions in the end.'

Another side to the harm caused by drugs is the excessive use of prescription (or even over-the-counter) remedies. Again, I can only mention that I hardly ever need nor take any of these unless I have a genuine disease! I am guessing that the majority of these potions are for pain relief, sleeping (and then as an adjunct - keeping awake) and depression. Unfortunately most of them have nasty and potentially dangerous side effects. I hope for those who are probably hooked on these helpers that you will find that many of the things mentioned in this book will allow you to overcome the habit. I also sincerely believe that following the advice in this book will ensure that most of you will never need to start taking such products regularly. Not surprisingly, many of the bad results are similar to those of illegal drugs and long term addiction to any form of medication, whether over-the-counter or prescription drugs, can lead to liver and kidney damage, and in some cases heart and blood pressure problems. With prescription stimulants for example, taking excessive doses could cause irregular heartbeat, distorted thinking leading to paranoia, heart failure, seizures, or even death. Unfortunately, just because they are prescribed by a doctor for a specific complaint doesn't mean they are safe overall. The adverse effects of steroids are all well documented. Their effect on aging includes muscle weakness, hardening of the arteries, arthritis, degeneration of joints, cataract formation and weakening of the bones. Cough and cold remedies are another category of product that is abused, particularly by teenagers (because they are cheap and easy to obtain). Some of the short and long-term effects include insomnia, heart palpitations, blackouts, seizures, delusions, and brain damage. Perhaps you are thinking that surely we are protected by various governmental organisations. Well, sadly an investigation by the Consumer Reports group in the U.S. of 12 common prescription drugs found that the side effects, such as kidney failure, bone deteriation, heart attack, stroke and cancer were undetected or underestimated when the FDA (Food and Drug Administration) approved their use.

So that brings us to alcohol. Taken to excess, of course, it can cause quite a variety of health problems especially liver damage. It certainly doesn't help in the youthful appearance stakes. In particular, its effects can be seen in the facial skin as well as the eyes and in a generally poor physical condition, often giving rise to an overall hunched, lethargic impression. Too much alcohol can also cause dehydration which can create fine facial lines. The biggest visible impact is probably the ruddy, aged complexion due to broken blood vessels just under the skin.

I thought that declarations like "I had such a great time last night I can't remember anything" were only pronounced by inexperienced youth after drinking binges but it seems that this juvenile behaviour is becoming more prevalent amongst older age groups also. I'm certainly no teetotaller but I've never drunk to the extent that I threw up and in fact I've never really had a hangover. Since I started a more healthy eating regime, I rarely drink alcohol. I certainly don't drink at all while partner dancing – it's pretty difficult and just too dangerous! As for driving under the influence of alcohol or drugs, well, if you want to die young …. The by-word seems to be to drink alcohol in moderation. Although generally too much alcohol has bad health effects, including difficulty in weight control, there are several studies which clearly show one benefit of alcohol – drinking one or two glasses of red wine a day can have a positive effect on cholesterol levels and blood pressure and may help protect against certain cancers and heart disease. However imbibing more than this amount apparently doesn't provide the benefits.

Review of Chapter 19

As expected, this chapter recounted the endless health and mental problems caused by the use of cigarettes, drugs and alcohol. These included the premature aging effects as well as early onset of illnesses and even death. Although there are likely to be times when we need to accept prescription drugs from a doctor, once again there were cautionary tales about the risks of abusing them. One faint positive glimmer was the fact that several studies have shown that moderate intakes of some alcohol, notably red wine, can have certain health benefits!

In Summary

If you have particular comments on any of the subjects in this book and especially some additional advice or success stories with any of the techniques, I would be very pleased to hear from you. If it seems useful to others then I would like to be able to consider acknowledging it in a future update of the book or on the website. See below for details of the email address and website location.

While it might be true that growing old is natural, looking old is optional; and hopefully you have found many ways in this book to work towards this alternative.

Different people define being healthy in various ways; they may concentrate on the need to be fit so the emphasis is on sports and exercise; some consider general well-being to be paramount and so focus on mental health and attitude. These are all well covered in this book. The other characterisation of good health of course, is having few illnesses. Personally, I rarely need to see a doctor. I have an occasional allergy to house-dust mites and when I lived in Sydney for a few years, I discovered that it was the haven of these microscopic monsters. A short series of injections soon fixed that! Apart from the sporadic tendency for my tonsils to become infected every five or six years, I just have no call for medical attention. Are you able to say that you only need to visit a doctor once every few years? If not then perhaps you should seriously consider taking action now and start working on the various techniques and approaches that I have described – many of them are important for your general health not just for youthfulness. You owe it to yourself, don't you?

Most people, by the age of thirty, and frequently younger, are starting to take note of the effects of age, especially on their faces. By the age of forty, the concern is often growing considerably. By fifty, many are becoming quite anxious about the ravages of time. In response, there are vast numbers of creams and potions all extolling their magical virtues and a susceptible public are buying stacks of them. Plastic surgery has seen an incredible surge in demand. However, certain of these procedures are at best only temporary and at worst have serious long term consequences and some are even miserable blunders causing actual mutilation. Many people, especially women are prepared to spend hours every week applying and cleaning off these products (which of course uses further special cleansing agents) or sitting in baths of the latest compounds in a desperate race against time. Almost as many spend huge sums every year having 'beauticians' apply the latest potions or exploit machines of all types on them. As consumers, we are spending billions of dollars a year on these industries.

Yet there are some very simple techniques that you can carry out on a regular basis that in most cases will work far better than all of the preceding activities put together. Moreover they cost nothing but a little time; probably less time than you are currently spending on rejuvenation right now. And surprisingly, they are all natural, healthy and safe. Don't you agree that they must be worth using? All it takes is to add a few practices into your daily routine or in most cases simply a change in some of your current habits.

In a nutshell these can be encapsulated by –

- Start carrying out the various activities outlined.
- Perform the specialised exercises described.
- Pay attention to your diet in the ways mentioned.
- Take note of the dress sense advice.
- Work on the mental attitude items.
- Practice the stress management techniques explained.
- Avoid certain items and behaviours that were detailed.

Perhaps for some of you, this seems like a daunting list but do not despair. One thing is for certain – you can read lots of books and attend seminars but this only gives you the appropriate information. Now you need to take action in order to benefit. Only you can decide, but don't you agree that it is worth taking action? Perhaps you might consider working on them one at a time until all those that you feel are relevant have eventually been taken on board. If you carry out only some of these items that I do then you too are likely to soon start looking years younger than your actual age. Best wishes with your future journey.

Email me at Derek@YearsYoungerNaturally.com

Visit the website at www.YearsYoungerNaturally.com

I will be gradually building up this website with more details on the subjects in this book and further information about areas of interest to my readers. Visit it regularly – put it in your 'Favorites'.